Love,
Jan

Love, Jan

A Personal Journal

Jan Bonn

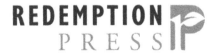

REDEMPTION PRESS

Republished by Redemption Press 2022. PO Box 427, Enumclaw, WA 98022.
Toll-Free (844) 2REDEEM (273-3336)

Unless otherwise noted, all Scriptures are taken from *Today's English Version* published for Catholic Extension by American Bible Society, 1966, 1971, 1976, New York. Used by permission.

Hard cover:
ISBN 13: 978-1-951310-71-4
Soft cover:
ISBN 13: 978-1-951310-70-7

Library of Congress Catalog Card Number: 2009908051

This book is lovingly dedicated to Hilary who allowed me freedom to write more than just the facts; to Tony who holds me when I cry; to Irene, Elizabeth, and Gabrielle who brighten my life; to Peggy who listens until I can figure things out; and to Debbie, Leslie, Julie, Susan, Amy, Sarah and the many friends who helped make this book a reality.

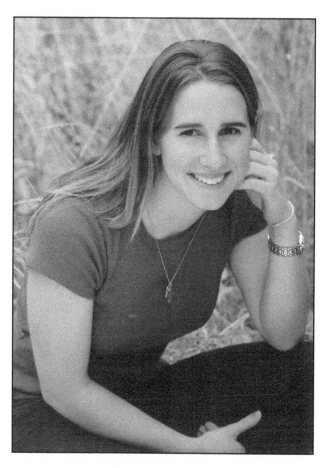

Hilary's Senior picture

Contents

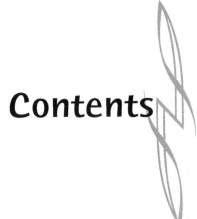

Chapter 3

Chapter 4

Chapter 5

Chapter 6

Introduction

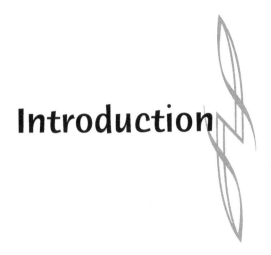

ON JUNE 25, 2002, our daughter, Hilary, was diagnosed with leukemia. To answer folks (people we love called family, and folks we know called neighbors) about Hilary's welfare, I started sending e-mail messages to everyone on our address list.

Most of these e-mails were sent from Portland, Oregon, where Hilary received treatment, but that's not where we're from. We live in a remote area of Oregon where the one-inch-thick phonebook contains the white pages and Yellow Pages of three counties and where we expect to travel at least one hundred miles to do any major shopping. I teach in Baker City at a school of three hundred students, and when I drive the forty-five miles to work, I pass more deer and nesting Canadian geese than I do cars.

Our town, a small agricultural town–or maybe now you would describe it as a small retirement or fishing town—in Eastern Oregon has seen some changes. The grade school has shrunk since I went to school there in the 'sixties, from around one hundred students in grades one through eight to fifteen students in June 2002. Now it is only open as a library and empty gym. We've seen some changes. Ours used to be the kind of town where people read the newspaper to check if the editor got the story right, because most of the time we already knew the story before the weekly newspaper arrived at our door. Now I read rather than hear the news.

We have space and scenery and animals, but it's the people who make the town. They are friendly, concerned, and loving. You can count on them to bring you food and feed your cows when you need help. Richland is a wonderful place to live.

Now let me introduce Hilary, our daughter. She was eighteen years old when she was first diagnosed and when I started writing the e-mails. I viewed her as a normal high school student, who spent her spare time running in track, playing basketball, training 4-H sheep, and singing with her sisters. She kept her hair long so people could distinguish her from Gabrielle, her identical twin sister. "Hilary hair" was her trademark. Her 5-feet, 2-inch slender frame held a confident, quick mind. Her bright brown eyes encouraged warm bantering. She was strong enough to wrestle a sheep and soft enough to cuddle a kitten. Hilary's welcoming spirit engaged and comforted those around her. Of course, Hilary would say I have a biased opinion.

She and Gabrielle had booked plane tickets for two days after their high school graduation to go to Alaska to work for the summer, but during the graduation ceremony Hilary was running a temperature. The fever didn't worry us as much as deciding whether or not to let her go as planned to Alaska. We asked the closest expert, a nurse practitioner from the health clinic in Halfway, for her advice. Because she couldn't see anything causing the fever, it seemed that a virus must be the culprit, and viruses don't last long in healthy, eighteen-year-old girls. Gabrielle promised to take good care of her sister. Plus, they were both going to work for Irene, their older sister, who I knew would be a kind, generous, and concerned employer. So, they packed their bags and flew to Illiamnia, Alaska, to work in a fishing lodge to earn money for college.

Sounds OK, doesn't it?

With Irene, Gabrielle, and Hilary in Alaska, my husband, Tony, and I were going to have a quiet summer. Elizabeth, our middle daughter, planned to paint houses for summer income. Tony, fix-it-man and first-rate father, was making plans to change his ranching lifestyle for a nursing career. Now that all the girls had graduated from high school, and having discovered that his volunteer EMT position provided a personal satisfaction that ranching didn't offer, he was ready to begin this new adventure. I wanted to start the summer with something exciting, so Grandma Bonn and I flew to Anchorage to visit Aunt Susan. Meanwhile in Illiamnia, Hilary wasn't getting over the virus. Because Irene knew I was in Anchorage, she flew Hilary there so I could take her to the doctor.

Grandma Bonn and I met Hilary's plane from Illiamnia, and we took her to a local health clinic. After three days of waiting for mono tests, we were advised to go to the emergency room for chest x-rays. It turned out that a virus was causing a horrible pneumonia. Hilary was moved to a room in ICU because her oxygen levels were at 82 instead of 100. I've always been amazed at the coincidence of Grandma Bonn and me traveling to Anchorage at that time. I call it a "God-thing"—a coincidence that God uses for our benefit. Some people call it a blessing. I have been forever grateful that I was able to be in Alaska to hold Hilary's necklace during her x-ray, take care of questions from nurses, and sit and watch her sleep when her temperature climbed.

When I called Tony that morning, he immediately left his ranching duties to neighbors, and caught the earliest flight he could find to Alaska. This required my brother, Wade, a day's drive away, to take Tony to Seattle to catch this flight.

After five days of many different tests and after being looked at by seven different doctors, it was discovered that leukemia had caused the pneumonia.

People have asked why it took so long to discover the evil enemy, acute myeloid leukemia (AML). Was the Alaska medical staff incompetent? The answer is no. The many nurses and doctors we saw were absolutely wonderful, professional people. Hilary's AML cells were gathering in her lungs, instead of floating along in her blood stream. Her illness presented itself as a wicked virus attacking her respiratory system, not a circulatory/immune system weakness, and only after a bone marrow biopsy was this evil enemy named.

The night before Hilary and Tony flew to Portland, the staff broke the ICU visitation rules and let Irene, Gabrielle, Grandma, Aunt Susan, and Tony and me visit with Hilary all at once—none of this one or two people at a time. We were all together and laughed too loud about hairstyles for Hilary after chemotherapy or silly hat ideas to cover a bald head; the nurses just shut the doors. When Grandma and I were getting ready for our own flight home, Hilary's nurse ran down to the waiting room to send us off with words of encouragement and a hug good-bye. They were wonderful! In the face of the unknown, the fear and terrible upheaval of life-threatening illness, the consideration and kindness of everyone in Alaska was a blessing.

Hilary was intubated for life flight and flown to Portland, Oregon. She was admitted to an ICU room at Oregon Health & Science University (OHSU). From there she got a room on 5C, on the oncology floor. And that's when I started this e-mail journal.

I wrote e-mails to my family and friends because they loved us. In turn, writing became an important tool for me to clear my rambling thoughts, and e-mail strengthened my connection to our wonderful small community and our family at large. Writing became for me an expression of prayer. E-mails asked other people to pray, when the best prayer I could muster was "Heal Hilary," and e-mails begged people to pray when in my anguish I couldn't. Once, after a night of helping Elizabeth watch Hilary suffer the distressing intubation tube at OHSU, I remember finding a solitary corner where I cried a demand to God, "Either heal her or take her to your home *this day*."

Of course, anyone who has suffered a long illness can tell their own story of turmoil. What makes our story different? Nothing. But some of the family and friends who received the "Hilary Updates" thought these letters could help other people in crisis. I'm praying this is so, that whoever reads this book will come closer to Jesus, the source of peace that passes all understanding, our healer of turmoil, fears, and tears.

                         Love,
                         Jan

Chapter 1

At Least We Know What We Are Fighting!

From: Jan Bonn
To: Everyone on our email list
Subject: Hilary update, day 4
Date: Tuesday, 25 June 2002

I'm sending this to everyone on our e-mail list. As all of you know, Hilary was diagnosed with leukemia last Thursday. We are now at OHSU in Portland. Her pneumonia is finally getting better. I'm hoping that she will be off oxygen soon!

The pneumonia is what caused us to go to the hospital in the first place, and then it took a few days to discover that this unusual-looking pneumonia was really leukemia. We felt the doctors and nurses in Anchorage were excellent, and the doctors here at OHSU told us we have not lost any time in our treatment.

The leukemia was hidden in the bone marrow and did not show its ugly head until the bone marrow aspiration revealed AML. Doctors were certain the pneumonia was a virus of some sort and were not eager to do any invasive tests to threaten an already weakened body. So, just as soon as they knew we were fighting leukemia, and not a viral pneumonia, Hilary was flown down in a hospital Learjet to Portland. Tony got to fly along with two nurses, the pilot, and Hilary.

After five days in the ICU, we moved to the floor for bone marrow transplant patients. We were given a room here because it is quieter and Hilary was so sick. She took her first shower yesterday, instead of a bath in a bed, and normal life feels sooooo good. She is still hooked to oxygen and has started chemo, but all the other tubes are gone. Yea, God!

We are not sure of all the steps needed for treatment yet. It is a hurry-up-and-wait game. After the first seven days of chemo, we wait for seven days then undergo another bone marrow test to see what the chemo has done to the leukemia. Then we decide what to do next.

The doctors seem excited that Hilary has a good chance of remission and cure. Many things are in her favor. One of those many things is your prayers and support. We feel God's love in this situation and feel your love and concern. Thank you. Hilary has never been frightened or worried about her illness. She is confident she will be cured and live a long life.

I hope this rambling note helps you understand a little of what we are doing and feeling. As soon as they put Hilary on an oxygen tank instead of being tethered to a hose that only reaches the bathroom, she can come down to this computer and write her own messages.

Thanks for all the prayers. God is in control!

Love,
Jan

WONDERFUL E-MAIL!

Hilary update, day 5
Wednesday, 26 June 2002

Wow, e-mail is a wonderful thing. I sent out one letter yesterday and received eighteen replies today, some which were from people who had received a forwarded e-mail from someone on my address list. It is so nice to be able to write one letter and have many people receive it at once. Just wanted you to know how grateful we are of all your prayers. I'm confident that those prayers are making this ordeal calm. Know that "peace that passes understanding" is in full bloom here.

Today Hilary is off oxygen and is walking down the hall with her IV pole and bags of fluids/drugs. Les, a guy who is going home soon, said, "Good for you, Hilary, for getting out. Let me give you my pole with a handle, because I won't need it anymore and you can move this pole so much easier."

Another guy named Mark poked his head out the door and said, "Hey, is that Hilary cruising down the hall?"

They both are praying for Hilary, and so we are praying for them as well as the other patients on this floor.

Today we went for a walk up to the sky bridge. The sky bridge is a marvelous structure. We think it is a fourth of a mile stretching between OHSU and Veterans Administration (VA) hospital. It is totally enclosed with windows all the way across. People can see the river and parts of the city. Maybe in a better spot, we can see Mt Hood. Of course, Hilary had on a mask and she was pushing her pole. Still, it is nice to see more of the world than walls.

We are starting to put up all the cards she is getting. Maybe we'll cover one full wall before we leave. Thanks again for all your support.

We love you,

Jan

Love, Jan

LEUKEMIA CHESS GAME

Hilary update, day 6
Thursday, 27 June 2002

Thank you for all the e-mails. I've read all of them to Hilary. It's nice to hear the news from home. When she found out that it has been over 100 degrees there, Hilary said, "I'm glad I'm here and out of that heat."

Some of you have asked about Gabrielle (Hilary's twin) and Irene (my oldest). They came to the hospital the night before Hilary left Anchorage and watched her get on the plane for Portland. Irene had her blood taken in Alaska to see if she was a matching donor for bone marrow, and then she flew back to Illiamna to go back to work. We call her daily to keep her updated, since she doesn't have access to e-mail up there.

Gabrielle came to Portland for her blood tests to check on being a bone marrow donor and left yesterday to go back to work. Irene will be glad to have her back. We won't know the results of those tests until sometime next week. Hilary has been told that she has a fifty-fifty chance of needing a bone marrow transplant.

I see this leukemia like a chess game. We made our first move, now we wait for the cancer to take its turn. Then it's our move. It takes strategy and wisdom. We need to look to the Creator of the universe for His wisdom to know the path. I think of Proverbs 3:4–5 (I think that is the Scripture that talks about him showing us the path to take if we will trust him. I know it is on a poster down in the basement of the Christian Church.)

Update: Hilary got her hair cut last night by Aunt Margaret's neighbor, who is an excellent beautician. They came to the hospital, and Shannon (the beautician) will take care of all the doings to send Hilary's hair to Locks of Love. She said it takes three ponytails to make one wig. Then she trimmed Hilary up so she is beautiful. In fact, I'm

4

amazed at how much she looks like Gabrielle with her short hair. They also brought Hilary some fish slippers that Lizzy couldn't wear. Hilary is smiled at by all who pass her. All the nurses think she is so cute, and many have gotten their picture taken by the wonderful squirt-gun camera that Tami Thompson brought her. She is bringing smiles to many on the floor. Well, I'd better close.

Love to you all,

Jan

HOW DO WE FIGHT?

Hilary update, day 7
Friday, 28 June 2002

We are getting so many encouraging notes—it is very nice. Today I read them and will report them to Hilary. The computer is in a room down the hall from her room and she was falling asleep in the chair. Being very tired is a normal response to the chemo she is taking. Other than being tired and her skin itching, she is doing great. She said she was a little queasy last night but no major nausea. The meds they use are wonderful for making this chemo as pain-free as possible. One guy said the worst part of chemo and this floor is boredom.

Yesterday, the doctors indicated that a bone marrow transplant might be the best way to fight this leukemia. We will know more after Hilary gets past this next week. The first step is remission. They have confirmed again that the pneumonia was probably caused by leukemia, which was stopping the blood from picking up oxygen. There has been no indication that the pneumonia was caused by virus, bacteria, or fungus, which is a good thing, now that her white cells are being killed by the chemo and she wouldn't have anything to fight off those kinds of intruders.

The nurses are encouraging Hilary to eat more and drink more water. She exercises when they offer her the opportunity, but her intake of nutrients needs to be higher. They are even bringing her candy bars, which she doesn't eat. The food tastes different because of the chemo (a little metallic), but her spirits are great and she never complains.

Thanks for the continued prayers. We appreciate them greatly. We see a few people here who don't have the support that you are giving us. I can't image fighting this disease alone. For a few days in Alaska I couldn't feel Jesus, and that was very uncomfortable. When Tony got there, I could relax and feel God's presence again. Having support is so important. Thanks for your prayers.

Love,

Jan

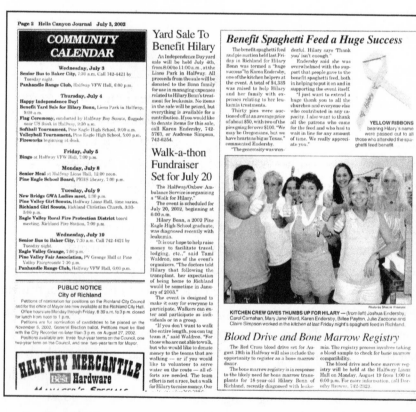

Spaghetti feed fundraiser was held at the Richland School. Grandpa Dad was overwhelmed with the generosity of our neighbors.

Donors

Hilary update, day 8
Saturday, 29 June 2002

We are so overwhelmed with your love for us! We have received a few e-mails about the spaghetti feed fundraiser held at the Richland Elementary School cafeteria. I'm not sure who coordinated this event, but Grandpa (Dad) said the place was packed with people from Richland and Halfway. We are overwhelmed with the outpouring of love. Hilary said she feels guilty. How does a person respond to such a showing of love? What does a person say? "Thank you" doesn't seem enough.

We have shared with a few people our goal to set up a bone marrow drive to add names to the national list of bone marrow donors. I have not been able to hook up with the Red Cross gentleman in charge of these things yet, but I have heard from other people in the bone marrow/ stem cell donor registry, who have said:

#1 It costs around $100 per person to be tested.

#2 The donors need to be between ages eighteen and fifty-five.

3 Younger donors are preferred because they can be on the list for a longer period of time.

4 The donors need to be healthy and willing to undergo the process of donating their bone marrow when needed.

I hope to have more information by Monday, and I will put Red Cross in touch with you guys over there. Hilary would like to donate some of the spaghetti-feed money toward this cause. Some of the people we have met use their own bone marrow to transplant[1] back into themselves, but anytime someone uses their own bone marrow, there is a higher chance of leukemia returning than from a matching donor. Anyway, this is the way we understand it. Irene and Elizabeth cannot be donors for Hilary even though this sister blood is so willing. Gabrielle is a matching donor, but we are waiting to see if she is an identical twin. If she is, there are some benefits and some problems. We are learning sooooo much. We will pass on to you things as we learn them.

We asked the doctors yesterday what a general timeline for Hilary would look like. We wanted to know when she can go home to Eastern Oregon. He thought probably we could plan on January 2003. Right now, they are saying a bone marrow transplant will be the path we will take. We will know more in a couple of weeks. We still need to wait until they do another bone marrow test on day 14 to make any long-term plans. I suppose I have confused many of you, because I am still so confused. Talk about a learning curve!

When Hilary and I prayed the Rosary yesterday, and we got to the part where we think about Jesus at age twelve visiting with the teachers in the temple, we prayed for wisdom about this disease and wisdom to see the path Hilary needs to take. We are confident that Jesus will light that path. Thanks again for all your love.

Thanks for eating spaghetti and buying pies. We pray to be good stewards of the money you are setting aside for us.

Love,
Jan

WASH HANDS

Hilary update, day 8, again
Sunday, 30 June 2002

Last night Hilary got her last bottle of chemo for the induction step. If she will eat and drink well, she can get unhooked from her IVs for a period of time. Today she ate some junk food (candy and nuts), and when her lunch came she didn't want to eat. Her stomach was upset, so junk food is now out. Really, we will all be healthier when this is over. We will eat better and wash our hands more often.

The nurses have told us that washing our hands eliminates most of the bacteria we would otherwise spread. Each time we enter the floor we must wash our hands for one minute.

Today, Hilary is getting a couple of units of red blood cells because her hematocrit is too low.[2] Other than that, she is doing wonderfully. Hilary looks, sounds, and feels very well. One visitor said if she didn't know Hilary was so sick, she'd think she was faking.

Thanks for all the prayers.

Love,

Jan

AUNT PEGGY

Hilary update, day 9
Monday, 01 July 2002

There is not much news today, but thought I'd better keep up the letter-writing. This will be a journal of this sorry adventure. Tony and Elizabeth headed toward Richland this morning, because Elizabeth needed to get some business finished at Eastern Oregon College. Elizabeth was not pleased about leaving Hilary.

Peggy, my sister, is staying with Hilary and me for a few days. We are reading, watching movies, trying to get Hilary to eat more (she weighed in at 99 pounds this morning), and resting. The only concern we have with Hilary right now is the calorie intake. She has no appetite, and so we are encouraging her to sip on Boost (a drink similar to Ensure).

While I was visiting with a volunteer from the Leukemia Society, Peggy worked out with Hilary during the exercise class. They both came back tired. It was nice to see the color in their cheeks. Thanks for all your encouraging e-mails. I love this form of communication.

Update on donor drive: I'm having trouble getting in touch with the person in charge of bone marrow drive donations at the Red Cross. Prospective donors may need to see what you can do in that area.

Talk to you tomorrow. Hope to send a picture then.

Love,

Jan

IDENTICAL TWIN?

Hilary update, day 10
Tuesday, 02 July 2002

It is now 6:00 P.M. and I'm just getting on the computer. Every time I tried earlier, someone else needed the room or the computer. Nothing new is really going on, but I knew that if I didn't write something, people would get worried. I remember when Irene was in South America, if I didn't get an e-mail often, I started to worry.

Hilary has slept most of the day, has not eaten much, but still has a great attitude. Peggy and I are starting to count her calories, just so she knows what her intake is. Today, she ate a few cashews and some ice cream. They tasted fairly good to her.

Yesterday she ate only 900 calories. We told her she needed at least 1000. She did ride the stationary bike for fifteen minutes, so she is trying to build her body. She says food just sits in her throat, so sips or small bites are the only way to go.

The news on the bone marrow donor program is: I've given it over to Dorothy Bower, who coordinates the blood drives for the Boise region of Red Cross in Halfway. The people at the Portland Red Cross have not responded to my questions, and I don't have the energy to pursue this.

Gabrielle is a bone marrow match for Hilary, but they are checking if she is an identical twin. If Gabrielle is an identical twin to Hilary, it would be too similar to an autologous transplant and the leukemia might return. If they find a perfect match that is not an identical twin, it might be a better solution. We will know more next week. Nevertheless, Hilary would like a few more names on the national bone marrow list for donors. This will help all the people who must use their own bone marrow because they can't find a matching donor. The more donors that are on the list, the better things are for all those in need.

When Hilary and I were praying the Rosary and thinking about Christ carrying the cross, it hit us that Simon was drafted into helping Jesus. That is exactly what you guys are doing. You are helping us carry this cross with all your support. We've had some wonderful visitors and great e-mails that make Hilary smile. Some of our family who live close to Portland have brought Tony, Elizabeth, and me suppers. We've had care packages of food, books, and movies. We've had offers of places to stay when the hospital time is up. (The doctors don't want Hilary to leave the area for a while even after she is released from the hospital.) All this and so much more. Thank you for helping us. Talk to you tomorrow.

Love,
Jan

SEAN

Hilary update, day 11
Wednesday, 03 July 2002

Well the computer froze up, and then it was busy, so it is after 9:00 P.M. and I'm giving my small update. (Since this computer is old and cantankerous, I asked the nurse to page Sean M., a former Richland neighbor from across the valley, who now works for the hospital in the computer department. He looked at it, but it still argues with us. I think it is just really old. Isn't it nice to have an important workman come and look at our stuff, just because he knows us? The nurse said she had to talk to Sean's secretary. Wow!) Now for the update:

Hilary had two bloody noses. They gave her platelets.[3] She started running a temperature (100.5) so they are doing some blood cultures, urine sample, and an x-ray of the lungs. She has a slight rash on the stomach, so they gave her some Benadryl, and she is sleeping. Her calorie intake was a little better today, she is working hard at eating. So...the day was not the best. We can only live one day at a time, so I'm glad that we have tomorrow to look forward to. I'm sure it will be better.

Love,
Jan

Low Counts

Hilary update, day 13
Thursday, 04 July 2002

Because Hilary will have a bone marrow biopsy[4] tomorrow, today has to be day 13. Today is a better day than yesterday. Hilary's temperature has stayed fairly normal and she is working hard to eat as much as she can. We planned to watch fireworks in Russ' room (he has a beautiful room that looks at Mt. Hood), but some of the nurses don't think the room is facing the right direction to see any fireworks. So, we thought that we could go to floor 14, to a waiting room that has windows all the way across. Hilary's nurse said, "I'm sorry Hilary, but your counts are too low[5] to leave the floor." I know that there are about four other patients who want to watch as well.

Ryan, (a twenty-three year old who came in two days after Hilary) stopped at Hilary's door and said, "I think we're all going to Russ' room for a July 4th look through his window."

So our plan is to wave a straw with one of the hospital's purple plastic gloves tied to it and watch what we can from Russ' window. We'll all have to wear masks, but oh well. I'll tell you tomorrow how it went. I've sure been thinking about the fireworks in Halfway, since we're trying to figure out a small celebration right here.

Have a great 4th of July! We'll be thinking of you.

Love,

Jan

4TH OF JULY

Hilary update, day 14
Friday, 05 July 2002

Below is a letter that Hilary sent out to her friends. I had her e-mail it to me so I could send it out to everyone on my address list. She is doing much better today. She still is working hard at eating, but her temperature was better today and she has had enough energy to check her e-mail. The best part of the 4th of July was the smile on Dale's face when he was pushing his pole down the hall, heading toward Russ' room, and I held up the straws with the gloves and told him they were our sparklers. He snorted and the nurses just smiled. I don't think Dale has laughed much. It was wonderful. The straws were Peggy's idea and the gloves were Debbie's idea. I'm the teacher who steals good ideas. Don't all teachers do that?

Enjoy Hilary's letter.

Love,

Jan

Hello, everyone,

I'm continuing to do well. I had a couple of days when I was really tired, but that's ok. I just slept a lot and didn't check my e-mail. That's why it's been so long since I've written. I'm back up to 102 lbs, so I'm gaining weight. It's hard though. My stomach can only handle so much. I'm not really nauseous, just really heavy feeling. I can feel every bite go down and sit at the bottom of my stomach. I drink a lot of high-calorie drinks, and that's where I get most of my nutrients. I'm just never hungry, and nothing tastes the same. It makes it hard. The 4th of July was fun. We went down to Russ' room (his room has the best view) to try and see the fireworks. We saw a lot that were going off in town. We didn't see very much of the big ones, but it was still a lot of fun. Mom made some "homemade" sparklers out of straws and the purple hospital gloves. I've kept mine so you can all see it when I get home. It was a fun day.

They took more bone marrow today to see if I need more chemo treatment. Doctor Maziars came back tonight and said the cells they saw looked different than the cells they saw when I first got here. So, that was very good news. They have to do more testing, so we'll know for sure on Monday if I'm going to need more chemo. The results were good enough today that they didn't have to start chemo tonight. I was happy about that. Well, I think that I'm ready to go take another nap. I'll talk to you all later.

Love,
Hilary

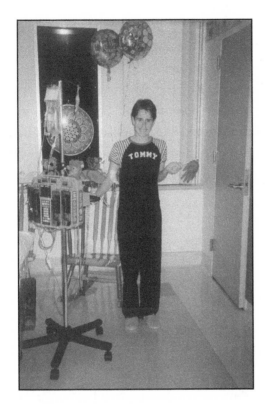

We had a great 4th of July celebration.

Love, Jan

BORING

Hilary update, day 15
Saturday, 06 July 2002

This was a very relaxing day. In fact the doctor said Hilary was boring. We like boring—no problems, major events, etc. I couldn't believe Hilary didn't tell the doctor that life could never be boring with Aunt Peggy and Mom around.

She had the nurse laughing this morning over her pills. The nurse didn't bring two fungus[6] prevention pills, because they were coming later. Hilary asked about them and told the nurse, "Actually, I hate those pills and don't really want to take them. I just thought I'd ask what happened."

Love you all lots. It is really nice to get letters that tell the news. Thanks.

Love,
Jan

COMPUTER MAN

Hilary, update days 16 and 17
Monday, 08 July 2002

Sunday. Sundays are always wonderful days. We had a few visitors, and then Ryan (the 22-year-old at the end of the hall) loaned us a movie that he thought was wonderful. Unfortunately, his mom needed to return it to Blockbuster that night, so we had to watch the movie as soon as possible. Thus I didn't get to the computer. So now it is Monday morning, writing about Sunday.

Hilary is still doing great. She is working on eating and writing a few thank-you notes. Aunt Shelly sent us some steak and mashed potatoes (with lots of butter added) and Hilary said they tasted pretty good.

16

As for Aunt Peggy and me, we had an adventure which will be in my memory for many years. It started with the Sunday *Oregonian*'s thrifty page. I saw an ad for a laptop computer for $200. Tony and I had planned to get Hilary and Gabrielle each a laptop computer for their graduation gifts, something they could use for college, and just hadn't started shopping yet.

Well, Peggy called and asked the guy what was wrong with the computer and he said, "Just because it is for sale doesn't mean there is something wrong with it."

He talked extremely slowly and she said he sounded like a computer nerd. Now explain to me, how can you tell a person is a computer nerd just by how they talk? Anyway, he promised to guarantee the computer for forty-five days after purchase (maybe it wasn't how he talked, but what he said), and Hilary said we could have Sean M. take a look at it. If it was bad, we would return it.

So off we went to the computer man. We drove up to this deserted house, no curtains in the windows, tall dead grass in the yard, and I told Peggy we must be at the wrong house. She said that we were to knock at the door to the right, not the front door.

The door on the right looked painted and possibly used, so we approached the door. I noticed a couple of boxes by the door that looked like garbage. Peggy rang the doorbell, prompting a wolf-like dog to begin barking and growling, as if in attack mode. With his head hanging over the edge of the flat roof, he seemed to be just inches from the tops of our heads.

I was confident that he was chained, but Peggy said, "He is not chained."

Debating whether to run for our lives or go for the good computer deal, our thrifty nature prevailed. Coming to our rescue was a 5-feet, 7-inches, 120-pound man in shorts, flip-flops, and T-shirt, smelling of body odor. Peggy asked if the dog (wild beast) was chained. The slow-talking, smelly little man said with little regard for our well-being that the dog had only jumped off the roof one time, and he had never done it since. Peggy wondered where the body is buried of the person who rang the door bell on that fateful day.

Entry into this computer maze showed why he had to be so thin. Peggy and I had to turn sideways to avoid the boxes, papers, and stuff stacked from floor to ceiling. Only with our backs against the wall to squeeze through the door, and turning right could we find the small stairway to his computer den. We were greeted by more piles of boxes and stuff at the head of the stairs. His two work areas were completely covered by stuff. The small kitchen in the back was completely covered by stuff. It smelled like body odor, wet dog, and moldy papers.

We discovered that this gentleman earned his living retrieving leased laptops from businesses that are upgrading their inventory. He then checked them out for problems and sold them. He seemed honest, even though he was dirty. He definitely knew his computers…so we bought the computer. When we got back into the car, both Peggy and I laughed for quite some time. It was like being in a movie. We wondered if this guy could possibly have a social life. Peggy then told me that he said on the phone that his dog would tell him when the doorbell rang. She'd assumed it would be a small yapping dog, not a wolf.

Of course, both of us would never have stayed if we had not had each other for protection and support. While I was asking questions, Peggy was thinking, *Jan, just buy it or not buy it. Don't talk, let's get out of here.* We, of course, showered before we walked back into the hospital. Who knows what kind of germs lurked in the corners of that place. What a memory!

Hilary wanted me to remove the loose hairs from her head. Well, after the removal, Hilary looks like a concentration camp survivor. Still, she is really cute. The short, sparse hair makes her eyes look huge, and she is beautiful! I think the hair loss bothered Peggy and me more than it did Hilary. We just reminded ourselves that Uncle Wade said, "If you lose your hair, it just says the chemo did what it is supposed to do. You want to be bald." When this morning she was down two pounds, Peggy said, "I didn't know hair was that heavy." Hilary didn't even laugh. She is so disappointed that she lost weight after working so hard at eating.

Today or tomorrow she will have a spinal tap to make sure there are no cancer cells in the spinal fluid. She will get some packed red blood cells today, because her counts are low, which they are supposed to be. She will probably leave the hospital within two weeks, and then they administer what they call consolidation chemotherapy.

Peggy and I have a couple of leads on some apartments. We have been offered places to stay, but I decided that we need a place to call home rather than using a bedroom in someone else's house. The hospital also insists that our place be within a twenty-minute drive of this place.

I'd better stop my rambling. I'll probably not write tonight. Talk to you again tomorrow. We know that God is in control of everything. Thanks for your prayers.

Love,

Jan

HEALING WITH MUSIC

Hilary update, day 19
Wednesday, 10 July 2002

Sorry I didn't write yesterday. I just didn't get to the computer room. Peggy left for Southern California at 11:30. She first took me to Josh and Chelsea Rohner's (my niece, Wade's daughter) house to borrow a car, so I would have transportation. Then she headed to the airport. It felt so quiet and lonely without her around.

At 12:30, Hilary got her spinal tap. It was uneventful! Praise God. The first results said no cancer in the spinal fluid. I'm confident that the final results will be the same. Hilary slept, I read, and then the evening was upon us.

Love, Jan

Today I moved out of the Ronald McDonald House. I'll sleep at the hospital, just like I've always done, and I can even shower here. I put some money down on an apartment. We can move in on Monday. Tony's family is loaning us furniture. Tony is planning to come back this weekend from Richland, but every time he plans to return, he is exposed to another bug. So, he sacrifices his desires of being here with us and numbly works irrigating pastures, mowing, bailing, and moving hay. Elizabeth is returning to work and will come whenever she gets a chance.

At 1:00 this afternoon, Dornbecker had a "healing with music" concert. It was a piano player. Hilary wanted to go and the doctors said OK. She rode in a wheelchair, wore a mask, and stayed in the fringes away from sick kids and enjoyed it very much. What a treat!

Well, it is 9:30 and I'm getting tired.

Love you all!
Jan

P.S. We read Psalm 91 this week and I'm trying to memorize the last part of it. It is really nice!

GABRIELLE IS AN IDENTICAL TWIN

Hilary update, day 21
Friday, 12 July 2002

Great news! Hilary might be able to leave the hospital by Monday or Tuesday if her neutrophil count reaches 500. I asked about day 28's bone marrow test and they said that could be done as an outpatient. She might even be able to come to Eastern Oregon for a couple of days around the 20th. That was great big news for me. I thought she wouldn't be able to come to Richland until after this was all over. We are very excited! They said they would need to teach us how to give IV antibiotic, and I thought future-nurse Tony will get great experience.

20

We found out yesterday that Gabrielle is an identical twin. So, as a donor she is not the first option, but the second. Yet we are so blessed to have her as a donor. I don't care if it is the second place. I just thought about Adam being God's first man creation, then after many years, he needed to send Jesus, his son, next to get us back on the right track. Maybe second is the best way to go!

Moving out of this room will take a truck. We have been blessed with many gifts. Just removing the cards off the walls will take a good fifteen minutes. My sister-in-law Mary Goin's doily sits on the windowsill and will be missed by the whole staff here. Every nurse has commented on how beautiful it is.

We love you all.

Jan

P.S. Please, all you walkers on the Hilary Walk: be careful. We don't want any heart attacks, heat strokes, etc. We heard how hot it was over there. Please be careful!

NEUTROPHIL COUNT

Hilary update, day 22
Saturday, 13 July 2002

When things start to improve, they move fast. Hilary's platelets[7] doubled yesterday, and her neutrophil count moved from 100 to 245. We are confident that she will be able to move to the apartment on Tuesday.

If you come to Portland, please come and visit. Hilary enjoys company. You will have to wash your hands and do no hugging, have no cold or flu virus, or no exposure to such things, etc. Even though she is able to leave the hospital, they give her many safety rules; like no crowds, no eating at restaurants, no fresh fruits, vegetables, or flowers.

Love, Jan

I hope to get as much in place as possible on Monday. I want to again thank all those people who offered us a place to stay. We chose an apartment mainly for two reasons: (1) the number of people who will be coming and going—we have a large family, and (2) we thought Hilary would be more comfortable in a place she could call her own.

Talk to you again tomorrow.

Love,

Jan

PICC LINE

Hilary update, day 23
Sunday, 14 July 2002

We started our day at 4:30 this morning. After Hilary went to the bathroom, she came back into the room and said, "Mom, my PICC line is coming out." For those of you who are wondering what a PICC line is:

PICC stands for peripherally inserted central catheter, which is an IV catheter in a large vein that travels to the right vena cava, so it empties into just above the right atrium (which is one of the four chambers of the heart). From this line, all chemo therapy, fluids, IV antibiotics, etc., can enter the body, plus the nurses can draw blood without a poke to the arm, hand, foot, etc. It is pain-free to insert once the first stick is finished—another great way to keep patients comfortable.

I could see 9 cm of extra line out of the arm. We of course told the nurse about it immediately. Then we waited until 6:30 for the IV therapist to look at it. Then we waited until 10:30 for the x-ray department to take pictures to find out where the end was. Apparently everything is OK. The dressing was changed and the line is now coiled under the bandage. Hilary is relieved that nothing needs to be done, but she is a bit worried about the safety of this line.

We've had some wonderful company yesterday and today. We're expecting Tony and Elizabeth later. That will be very nice! Visitors are the colored jelly beans in an oatmeal day.

After much discussion, we are not coming to Richland for our two-day respite. It is too far and too hot for such a short time. We are a bit disappointed, but everything comes in its proper time.

Well, I'd best go and see if Tony and Elizabeth are here yet.

Love to you all.

Jan

Chapter 2

APARTMENT

Hilary update, day 24
Tuesday, 16 July 2002

Good morning, everyone. Today is release day.

Yesterday, Hilary's neutraphil count was over 500 and her white cell count was over 3. I asked the doctor if we could stay one more day because even if Hilary's body was ready to leave, I was not ready to take her to the apartment. There is security in this womb-like hospital.

Ready or not, last night Mary (Tony's sister), Dale (her husband), Sarah (our niece), Mike (Tony's brother), and Katy (Mike's daughter) moved us in. They brought stuff from the attics and garages of sisters and brothers from Albany, Portland, and Springfield. We're expecting more later this week, but our place looks very homey and we are now ready for Hilary to "come home." It is so wonderful! We have a phone that works, so you can call us. A beautiful couch and loveseat, and table and chairs, and Mary even brought a box of food to stock the pantry. I walked around in circles, dazed at the beauty of it all.

Love, Jan

Hilary is still having headaches. We hope to have a blood patch, which was explained to me as a patch made of blood that will act like a Band-Aid to stop any leakage from the spine. Any loss of spinal fluid can cause headaches. Hopefully that will take care of the headache problem. Other than that, she is very well.

Thanks for all your letters. They are wonderful!

Love,

Jan

WATCH AND WAIT

Hilary update, day 28
Friday, 19 July 2002

I'm writing this update from Aunt Shelly and Uncle Mike's computer. We thought of using the library computer (it is only half a mile from our apartment), but the library was really busy and using public computers for Hilary is scary. Anyway, Shelly said to come and use their computer, so here we are. The laptop computer didn't work out. We sold it to Mark, another patient on the floor, who was confident he could handle all of its problems. I was glad not to have to visit the dog and his master to return the computer.

Now for a review of the last few days: Tuesday, Hilary had a blood patch for the headaches caused by the spinal tap. It seemed to help. Then we arrived at the apartment around 2:00. Hilary proceeded to vomit six times throughout the evening. I was very nervous, wondering why this was happening. Of course I called the clinic and was given directions to watch and wait.

Wednesday, was a very calm day. Everything seemed fine.

Thursday, Hilary started to run a temperature. I again called the clinic and we added another medicine to her list.

26

Today, we needed to visit the clinic for blood check, blood pressure, weight gain/loss, and a general looking over. Her blood counts are doing great. She had her bone marrow test and we will find out the results on Tuesday. This is the weekend we can leave town, and our plans are to go to visit relatives in Albany. If Hilary's temperature returns, we will stay in Portland. I don't handle unknown problems (like elevated temperatures) very well.

I had one interesting event happen on Tuesday before we left. Over a few days, we had been visiting with a fellow patient, who was around Hilary's age, in the computer room as we waited for our turn at the computer. He came in while I was writing, and I had a chance to mention that I noticed that he didn't seem to have any visitors. He told me his dad couldn't drive, and his mom worked all the time. I had to share about the wonders of our Christian family. I told of the wonderful couple in Alaska who came to the hospital ready to be Hilary's mom and dad because they thought she was all by herself. They found out about Hilary through a prayer request from Hilary's Aunt Susan. I hope he understands that if he wants a larger family, Christ's church is a wonderful place to look.

Hilary was watching me write this e-mail and she said, "Mom, say good-bye." I think she might be tired. Good-bye.

Love you all.

Jan

APARTMENT MANAGER

Hilary update, day 29
Saturday, 20 July 2002

We are again at Aunt Shelly's house. Our shower decided to plug up today and Tony headed back to Richland. The manager is not home right now to get my message about the shower, or there would probably

27

Love, Jan

be a plumber here. The manager is working very hard to keep our place in great working order. Her father died of cancer two years ago and she is very concerned about Hilary's safety. I am continually amazed at the kindness people show.

There is nothing left to say. Have fun during the walk (you crazy people who are walking thirteen miles in the hot weather). Take care of yourselves.

We love you!

Jan

Page 6 Hells Canyon Journal August 21, 2002

Walkathon Nets Thousands for Hilary

Photos courtesy of Pat Matheson

by Tami Waldron

The idea of the Hilary walk started the morning of the community prayer for Hilary in town. We were mulling over ideas to raise money for miscellaneous expenses that may arise during Hilary's treatment for leukemia, such as a spaghetti feed, yard sales and the like. The Halfway/Oxbow Ambulance Service wanted to do something special as well, and we came up with a sponsoring a walk, "Over the Hill for Hilary."

The event took place on Saturday, July 20. We began at 6:00 a.m. from the Halfway Ambulance Barn. The temperature was refreshing; the sun was up (barely), and we were off. As we walked over the hill, we saw various animals including coyotes, deer and elk. Those driving by gave us honks, waves and encouragement. The walk went from the Halfway Ambulance Barn to the Richland Ambulance Barn, encompassing a total of 13.3 miles.

The walkers represented Oxbow, Richland, Sparta and Halfway. They included Jackie Smith of Sparta; Carolyn Crawford, her daughter Karen Hank and grandson Tabor who was five months old (Tabor actually got to do the walk in his stroller); Evelyn Ruggles and Christine Bennett of Oxbow; Tami Waldron and her daughter, Stephanie Brown; Butch Michaelson; Lisa McCarthy; Shelley Welch; Ben Bishop; Anne Shields; Rachelle Robinette and her dog, Apache; Joey and Holly Gover; Jessie Godwin; Samantha Dyke and Dalton Stroud, both seven years old, of Halfway; Debbie Immoos; Laura Hale and her dog, Max; and Dave Clemens of Richland.

Those who walked from the Richland side gave pull down to the Richland Ambulance Barn were Sue McCleary and her daughter, Katie McCleary; Paula Story; Darlene Beam and her father-in-law, Martin Beam, who is 84 years old.

As we walked, two bicyclists went speeding by. They were Zan Bates and George Mattle, who rode their bikes from Carson to Richland.

Those who helped on the road included Dorothy Brower, Red Tarter and Jerry Welch. They provided transportation, water, fruit, and music at our stops. At the summit, Jerry had Willie Nelson singing "On the Road Again."

Carl Hintz, owner of Eagle Valley Sanitation, provided us with a truck and porta-potty. The consensus of the walkers was that it was the cleanest porta potty we'd ever been in. Fred Riggs was the chauffeur of the portable outhouse. At one point in the walk, one group had a cell phone and called down to Fred, summoning him up the hill.

Anne Shields got us in the recycling mode. She was picking up cans, and it wasn't long until we all were in the borrow pit, gathering cans. Stephanie provided us with laughter and videoed the event for Hilary. Delores Buskler refreshed the walkers and provided a homemade soup just as we came down into Richland.

We made far better time than we had planned. We were all over the hill and finished at 10:30 a.m.

And stay tuned for part two. Wayne Endersby promised that he would walk over the hill when he got home from the fire.

(Editor's note: Longtime Pine Valley resident Tami Waldron is a local business-woman and an EMT with the Halfway/Oxbow Ambulance Service. As of last Sunday, Tami said the walk, dubbed "Over the Hill for Hilary" had netted over $8,000 for Hilary Bunn and her family. The Journal extends its thanks to Tami for this write-up and to Pat Matheson, an Eagle Valley EMT, for use of the photos. Congratulations to everyone who participated in the walk, whether as a walker, a donor or in a support capacity.)

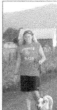

DANCING VIDEOGRAPHER – Stephanie Waldron Brown got off to an enthusiastic start for Hilary.

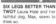

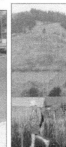

BEAUTIFUL MORNING FOR A STROLL – water bottle in hand, Jennifer Godwin walks the half-marathon-equivalent distance with a smile.

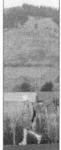

SIX LEGS BETTER THAN TWO? Laura Hale and her faithful dog, Max, seem to think so.

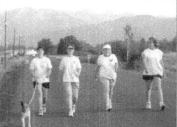

ROAD WARRIORS – (from left) Rachelle Robinette, with her dog, Apache, Lisa McCarthy, Shelley Welch and Tami Waldron.

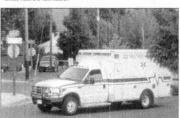

HIGH-TECH SAG WAGON – An ambulance paced the walkers just in case, and to pick up anyone who found the grueling 13-mile walk too challenging.

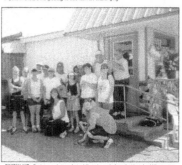

FINISH LINE – Footsore and weary, but exhilarated nonetheless, the triumphant hikers relax in the shade at teh Cappucino Corral in Richland.

ANNE SHIELDS appears unchallenged as she begins the walk on Main Street in Halfway.

DAY-HIKING – Dave Clemens of Richland walks briskly down the road

Thank You

On behalf of the Halfway/Oxbow Ambulance Service we want to take this opportunity to thank all of you who supported this effort in any way. As of Sunday, August 18, we have in hand just over $8,000.00.

A special thanks to everyone who came out and walked, and those who helped provide support for the walkers while they were going over the hill.

There was also plenty of behind-the-scenes support from people who didn't make the walk. Supporters included the Methodist Church in Richland, and especially Isle Gravers, specifically for bookkeeping the pledges; Old Pine Market provided our coolers with ice; Karen Endersby made the "Caution Walkers" posters and Wayne Endersby made the pledge sheets; Pat Matheson and Pearl Duman provided the water and encouragement to those who started the walk on the Richland side, as well as those who came over from Halfway; The Grange and Richland Ambulance Service were willing to open up their buildings to us as well; Artesian Blue Water Company from Cove, Oregon, donated cases of water, and Safeway donated cups.

Because of each of you, this WalkOver the Hill for Hilary was an overwhelming success.

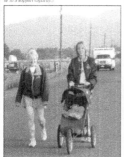

THREE GENERATIONS OF CRAWFORDS – Carolyn Crawford of Brownlee (left) walks with her daughter, Karen Hank, and Karen's son, Tabor, who was the only child to go over the hill in a stroller during the fundraising walk.

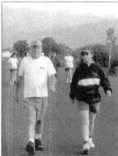

ALL LOCAL COMMUNITIES REPRESENTED – Butch Michaelson of Halfway and Debbie Immoos of Richland walk closely in the early going of the 13.5-mile route. Hikers from Sparta, Oxbow and Brownlee also joined the walk for a worthy cause.

Chapter 3

BELOVED OF CHRIST

Hilary update, day 33
Wednesday, 24 July 2002

Welcome home—I'm back at the hospital computer. The results of Friday's bone marrow biopsy were good and bad. Hilary is in remission, but she had some suspicious-looking cells. Instead of a three-day outpatient chemo, she has a five-day in-hospital patient chemo. She was not excited about being back in the hospital, but she is not a complainer.

This is just the next step in the process to getting well. We hope to be back in our apartment directly after the chemo. Unfortunately for this mom/caregiver, I know that it is the week after chemo that is the hardest. As much as Hilary likes visitors, we can only accept a few. Please be sure to call first. If Tony had his way, Hilary would not have any visitors. We heard that the "Hilary Walk" was very successful. Thank you for all your effort and sore muscles. We are looking forward to seeing the video.

For those of you who asked about our plumbing: yes, our tub is working fine. We have no more leaks or plugs. Praise God! We had a wonderful visit in Albany. If we couldn't go home to Richland, Albany is a great second choice. We visited with aunts, uncles, cousins, and Grandma Bonn.

There were lots of laughs and great food. What else can make for a great time but lots of laughs and great food! We love you all! God's blessings to you all. Did you know that you are Christ's beloved? Mark, a patient we met on 5C, calls Hilary "Beloved of Christ." Has a nice ring to it, doesn't it? You also fit that description.

Love,
Jan

ONE DAY AT A TIME

Hilary update, day 34
Thursday, 25 July 2002

Hilary is doing very well. She is sleeping a great deal, which is good. Because her counts are still high, between her naps we went for a walk outside and on the sky bridge today. You can see the Willamette River, a bridge across the river, and trees, boats, cars, tables and chairs from a restaurant, plus all kinds of people.

Last night was interesting. We are on 5A instead of 5C, so each room has the possibility of being shared. Hilary is not sick enough (Praise God) to be on 5C this time. Anyway, I was sleeping in the other bed when at midnight the nurse came in and said he was sorry, but they needed that bed. They got me a cot and we were settled when the other patient arrived. She was very loud about giving directions for eliminating her pain, plus loud cries when she felt pain. As soon as they had her in place, they proceeded to move us to another room so we could get some rest. We shared the next room with a wonderful lady who was just diagnosed with a very rare form of cancer. She'd had surgery and was released today. I could sense the fear from her daughter—that fear of the unknown.

32

I also met a lady whose son has a rare form of liver cancer. They are here for a surgery on his pelvis, just stealing time, in hopes that the research will provide some answers before the cancer takes his life. She was a woman of faith and stated again, "We can only live one day at a time. We make the most of each day we are given." Amen.

After meeting some of these people, I feel so blessed with the cancer we are battling. Leukemia research has made such gains that we have more hope than these people. Yet, we all live one day at a time and we need to make the most of each day we are given. Amen.

Love to you all.

Jan

GIFTS FROM HOME

Hilary update, day 35
Friday, 26 July 2002

We had a very nice surprise last night. Mark (my principal in Baker) and his wife, Patty, and daughters, came with four sacks of gifts from various people in Baker. He and his family were on a short vacation visiting the Portland area and they made a few phone calls to see if anyone wanted to send some greetings. Such wonderful greetings! We are always overwhelmed with the generosity of our Eastern Oregon neighbors! After Mark and Patty left, Tony and Elizabeth popped in. It is always nice to have everyone around.

Today has been a boring day. Boring days are good days! Hilary has slept a great deal. Elizabeth and I did a few things at the apartment while Tony stayed and watched Hilary sleep. We then went for our daily walk and visited with some friends on floor 5C.

Talk to you again tomorrow. God's blessings!

Love,

Jan

Love, Jan

KNOW YOUR LIMITS

Hilary update, day 36
Saturday, 27 July 2002

Today we had a new PICC line put in. The old one just kept working its way out. We're hoping that this one will last for the duration of all Hilary's treatments. I've noticed that this hospital has a "no pain treatment" whenever possible. They make each day as comfortable as they can. They want Hilary to exercise and stretch, but be smart and not go too far. She needs to remember how far it is back to her room and to know her limits. Isn't that good advice for all of us. What a fine line it is to know when to push and when to stop! I can't believe that it was only a week ago that many of you pushed (walked) your way over the hill. Thank you again.

Talk to you tomorrow, and love to you all,

Jan

PONDERING HEALING PRAYERS

Hilary update, day 37
Sunday, 28 July 2002

Sunday and we didn't make it to church. We tried, but folding clothes took longer than planned. We knew the church here would not wait for us like you folks at home, so we stayed at the apartment.

Then my cousin Linda called about seeing if some people from her church could come and pray with Hilary. That prompted me to think again about prayers and healing.

Question: Why are some people healed, and some are not, when we pray for healing?

I know that in the past I've prayed to Jesus with the same attitude I've had when I've asked for a gift—hopeful, but not believing.

I've also prayed "I claim this in Jesus' name," but this seems to be a demanding attitude. Who is in control? Us or God? Do we trust God to love us beyond what we think is right?

During my college years, I was taught that sickness is a consequence of sin; therefore when illness comes about, it is evidence that a sin was committed. This created a guilty attitude, which in my case was neither healthy nor correct. I've read in the gospels that sometimes sickness is to glorify God.

During one luncheon date with Sandra Traw, she mentioned that she believed that God always tells us who will be healed in body, so we know how to pray. This is communication when we listen to Jesus speak to us. This is faith. This is what I want. Every situation is different, and I want a God that deals with me in a customized manner—just for me. Not a formula.

I've also been told that when Jesus was beaten, it was through the stripes on his skin that we are healed. Isaiah 53:4–5 supports the idea of healing because of Jesus' stripes. This makes me cry to know how much Jesus suffered so we can be healed.

Enough philosophy!

Hilary will have her last chemo tomorrow morning, and then we will be back in the apartment. Her counts should drop for a week or so, and then they will start back up. Twenty-eight days from now they will take another bone marrow test and then we will take our next step.

Eating is starting to become hard again. Everything tastes funny, but she knows what she needs to do and is already working at keeping her calories and fluids at a good number. She does not have nausea, mouth sores, or any other problems. Praise God.

I'll visit again when I get the chance.

Love,

Jan

Love, Jan

SANDRA'S LETTER

Hilary update, Fwd: Healing
Monday, 29 July 2002

Sandra is a cousin of mine who is also a nurse. I asked if I could forward her response to my e-mail about healing and prayer. Enjoy.

Love,

Jan

Jan,

I had totally forgotten about visiting with you on the healing issue. I went through a huge struggle with regard to the issues surrounding healing. I had seen so much that I did not understand, and for that matter I still don't. But for me it was important that I come to grips with what I really did not believe. I saw people with great faith not healed and people with no faith healed. I also became convinced that it had little to do with sin in our lives. It never did "feel right" when I tried the authority thing…the claiming thing seemed pretty lazy to me. If God did not miraculously heal you of a broken leg, it seemed a little hard to walk around saying, "I've been healed" when the leg remained broken. Or to go around without your glasses claiming restored vision when you were walking into walls.

Yet, if it was not God's will to heal, how could I be a nurse trying to heal people? What if God didn't want people cured of their headache and I was giving them pain medication? What if he wanted them to suffer so that they would be more spiritual? What a struggle I had with the whole issue. All I really knew was God's nature by looking at Jesus' work on earth. He had great compassion and healed most if not all who came to him. Although the Bible did say he was unable to perform miracles in one place because of the unbelief.

36

Then Raquel got stress fractures the full length of both tibias and was in so much pain she was unable to play ball that year. She wanted prayer to be healed. As I started calling people to pray for her, the standard answers that I got were things like: God has something better for her than to play ball. God does not always heal because he as a lesson for us to learn. By the time I had finished calling ten people, I was depressed and very confused. Even the people I considered men and women of faith gave the same answers. No one said, "Sure I'll pray." They first gave me all the reasons that God might not heal. I never will forget what happened when I told Raquel some of the answers that I had gotten. She said "Mom, I love the Lord and if he didn't want me to play ball all he had to do was tell me. He didn't have to give me stress fractures and I don't believe he did, no matter what they say."

I thought, "This is getting serious and I have no answer." I spent days in the Scriptures seeking an answer. The Lord kept taking me to Paul's prayer for the thorn to be removed. The Lord kept asking me how long Paul prayed and I kept saying three times. Does this mean we pray three times and then stop? I knew in my spirit that I was not getting what the Lord was trying to tell me. I read day after day, and still nothing. I finally started fasting and God kept asking me the same question. How long did Paul pray? How long did Paul pray? Finally one day I heard an answer so clear that I thought it had been spoken aloud: *"Paul prayed until I spoke!"* That was the answer I had been looking for. He said, *"I just happened to speak on the third time. Sometimes I speak sooner, sometimes it is much longer, but keep praying and believing it is my desire to heal until I speak and say my grace is sufficient."*

I thought back to the many times that had been true in my life. I remembered when Grandma Honey was very ill from a fall and I was praying for her healing; I felt the Lord was saying to me *"I will heal her now, but the next time do not pray for her healing."* I told my sister Glenda what I felt the Lord had said. We celebrated Christmas that year believing it would be Grandma Honey's last one with us. When she had her heart attack the following May, I was not able to pray for her healing but prayed for her to not fear and to be at peace. The last thing she said to my mom was, "Donna, I'm going and you need to accept it."

I thought about how bad I had felt when I could not pray for Jane to be healed. From the very start I felt God was going to take her home. I felt so guilty about not having faith. Now I understood he was saying, *"My grace is sufficient for Jane."*

So now I keep praying for healing, believing it is God's will to heal. Until he speaks to say otherwise—and believing that he will speak to me as he spoke to Paul, and if we stay open to hear his voice, he will tell us to stop praying for healing and begin praying for grace.

So it really isn't that he will tell us what he is going to do. There can be a couple of prayers when we hear, or it can be months or years, but he wants us to keep praying until "HE SPEAKS." And so it is that I continue to pray for Hilary's healing, believing with all my heart that he wants us to continue our prayers, and knowing that even through this hard time he has great gifts for all of you.

Oh, by the way, Raquel suffered much of the rest of that year, but the next year she made all-league volleyball, all-conference basketball, and her legs were strong enough for her to do track, which she had never been able to do because her legs were so bad. She went to district in the 200 and the short and long relays. We'll never know what would have been if we had stopped praying. I have a feeling that old saying "Don't stop praying five minutes before the miracle" may be more true than we know.

Sandra S Traw, RN

P.S. I don't mind others hearing what I believe the Lord told me, as long as they know that I don't claim to have "the answer." I believe that we only see and hear a glimpse of the full truth. I'm sure we will never be able to understand the full TRUTH in this life.

Chapter 4

GIVE US THIS DAY OUR DAILY BREAD

Hilary update, day 39
Tuesday, 30 July 2002

Yesterday we finished up the second chemo and came back to the apartment.

Today I made bread, creating pleasant food smells that say "Home." Hilary slept and watched me make bread. Tony went to Richland for a couple of days. Life is boring! Praise God!

The doctor indicated that we will plan for the transplant at the end of August. This is much sooner than we were first told. This is exciting news because the sooner we do the transplant, the sooner we see Richland and home.

Pretty exciting!

Love,

Jan

Love, Jan

VACATION AT THE CLINIC

Hilary update, day 41/day 8
Thursday, 02 August 2002

The clinic calls this day 8, because they count from Hilary's last chemo day. We went to clinic today and it was an experience. First they took blood to check all the blood numbers. Hilary's numbers are dropping as they should. They expect the lowest numbers to happen seven to ten days after chemo and stay low for about a week. We are planning very calm days next week.

Then a massage therapist asked if she could massage Hilary's hands and feet. She was from Florida and came to the Portland area to study under a specialist in cancer massage. She has since moved here with her husband and is hoping that the winters will not be too dreary. After that, one of the nurses and a patient played some jazz. The nurse played the ukulele and the patient played the trombone. An older gentleman who loves jazz wheeled in to join the couple. He was on floor 5C when we were there, and it was the first time I had seen him smile. We all laughed and especially enjoyed the port-a-potty song. We asked if this entertainment was normal, and of course it is not. Still, what a special day! It was like we were on vacation.

I read in the *Hells Canyon Journal* about the August 19th day for giving blood for the Red Cross. I hope many names are added to the bone marrow national list. Because Tony's sister Mary gives blood often with the Red Cross here in Portland, she is working on a "Hilary Bonn Party" to increase awareness of the need for blood donors. It is scheduled for August 31. We are hoping for some publicity to get the word out. Please pray for the success of this drive as we will pray for the success of your blood drive. If you are in the Portland area on August 31 and let me know, we'll get you set up down here. Dorothy, please advertise in Baker. Maybe some people from there would take time from their busy day to give a little blood so they can be typed for the national registry.

40

An update on the computer story: Because the famous laptop from the dog man needed parts I was unable to get, I sold it to Mark (a patient down the hall) for the same amount we paid. He knew of all the problems and was confident that he could get them fixed with little effort. Mark e-mailed me and said it needed a battery. I gave him the name and number of Dennis, the dog man, and they tried to call. No answer. Finally, they went over to the house and again no answer to the door, but the dog was there. When Mark called the computer man by name, he came out onto the roof of the garage and took care of their problem. I think that laptop has a happy ending. We are using a computer from Bob, Aunt Margaret's neighbor. It is working great. It is nice to have a computer at the apartment. I'd better close.

Love to all of you, and God's blessings.

Jan

BLACKBERRIES

Hilary update, day 44/day 1
Sunday, 04 August 2002

This is my second attempt at typing this letter. I had the whole thing finished and then my computer froze up and I lost it all.

We are doing great over here. We go to clinic again tomorrow and I'm sure that they will say, "Keep being boring." Wouldn't it be great if we had a massage person and some music again?

Tony got here Friday. He would rather be here than in Richland. His "protect family" personality can't do a proficient job when he is 300 miles away. The ranch isn't important when it demands time away from being here. Having Tony in our apartment certainly makes it more like home. He, Uncle Mike, and Katie picked some blackberries just outside our door yesterday. Then last night we made some pies. Even Hilary had a nice-sized piece with some ice cream. I was surprised because sweets have not been an eating choice for her.

Yesterday morning, Hilary and I went to the farmers' market just two blocks from our apartment. Hilary wore her duck mask, and I didn't notice people looking at her strangely. Maybe because our society is used to seeing purple hair, tattoos, and piercings, any attire is OK. Anyway, we bought some green beans, peas, a couple of nectarines, and looked at some quilts, and then we sat in a chair under an umbrella and listened to a musical group with a bass, guitar, piano, fiddle, and a female lead singer. I enjoyed watching a very old man stand close to the lead singer, tap his toe, and thoroughly enjoy the music. I considered asking him to dance, since he obviously enjoyed music, but I was afraid he might die of a heart attack or something worse. Really, I was afraid that he would refuse me. I remember all those days in high school when I sat along the side of the room waiting for someone to ask me to dance. It is awful being a wallflower. I'm so glad that today's youth dance in groups doing line dances or circle dances. Anyone can enjoy themselves at a dance.

Tony and I went to church today. It took us only ten minutes to walk. I think that is wonderful. When we said, "It is right to give you (God/Jesus) thanks and praise," I thought of all of you. I thank God/Jesus for all of you. You are so special.

Love,

Jan

P.S. I'm going to send this now. If it doesn't work, sorry—no letter today.

MOVIES TO PASS THE TIME

Hilary update, day 40-something
Wednesday, 07 August 2002

I'm losing track of time. Monday's clinic was long. Hilary needed two units of red blood cells and one unit of platelets. It took all day. Monday morning, she was so pale that I was not surprised at her low counts. Because her counts were so low, we are back to clinic today to check the numbers again. We bring reading material, and stuff to eat and drink, and plan to stay a long time. I'm using a computer in the corner that patients can use while they are waiting. Hilary is doing very well, but I'm glad they keep close track of those blood numbers and give her units when she needs them.

Yesterday my Dad and Phyllis came to visit. Phyllis had an appointment at the eye clinic. I'm so glad that they had a reason to come this direction; it was very nice to visit with them. They were so concerned about bringing Hilary some unwanted or dangerous bug. I appreciate their concern, but I'm so glad they came. Boring is a very good thing, but boring is, as they say, boring.

Last night we watched a G-rated movie called *The Basket*. It was very good. We thought of all you basketball players. It was set in Washington state during WWI. Basketball was just starting. I didn't remember that the teams used to jump in the center after every basket. The high score of 20 was a lot. I rented it at Blockbuster, only two blocks from our apartment. Hilary said I did a good job on that one. Check it out, you basketball players. Let us know of any movie titles that you think are worth watching. We've watched a lot of movies, so giving us a new title would be like trying to buy a gift for someone who has everything.

The nurse just came and said the labs look good. I'm sure that we'll get to see Susan, the nurse practitioner, soon and then we'll get to go. Love to you all! Stay boring. Enjoy the cool weather.

God's blessings upon your day.

Jan

APHERESIS

Hilary update
Friday, 09 August 2002

We are at clinic again today and Hilary needs some blood products. Thus, we've been here three hours and plan to be here at least another three. Even though we wait a long time, we have visited with many of the friends we made while on floor 5C. It is reunion time. We met a lady who has been told about Market America's aloe from a friend and wondered if we took it. (She saw the Market America emblem on a box I was planning to mail to Irene.) We told her that we thought the aloe was certainly not hurting Hilary, and in fact it might be one of the reasons she was doing so well. Aloe and prayer make a wonderful combination.

We have more information about the Hilary Bonn Party at the Red Cross, scheduled for August 31. First, the party is an apheresis party. Apheresis is the process of separating the blood into components such as platelets, which stop bleeding, or red blood cells, which carry oxygen. One friend says the process is very expensive. According to her, platelets are gold. Aunt Mary and Aunt Margaret are apheresis donors for platelets at least once a month. Platelets only circulate in the body for around ten days, so the Red Cross only keeps platelets for five days. They need willing platelet donors often. This "Hilary Party" will hopefully increase the platelet donor list and increase awareness. Second, this process takes about two hours. They give the donor juice, cookies, cake, and even a choice of movie to watch while passing the time. Third, we've been told that if a person is an apheresis donor three times, they can be added to the list of bone marrow donors for free (which is a savings of around $100).

Last! We are hoping to fill the Red Cross on August 31 for the Hilary Party. If you live in the Portland area or want to be a part of this party, please call Shirley at the Red Cross before August 15. Tell her that you need information about the "Hilary Bonn Party" and want to be a donor on that day. I'm hoping that we overwhelm them with people!

Well, they just told us that Hilary's red blood cells won't be here for another forty-five minutes. I think we will be here until 7:00 tonight. She wants to go check on Ryan while we wait, so I'd better close.

Love to you all,

Jan

STAYING BORED

Hilary update, day 52/day 19
Monday, 12 August 2002

We are boring. Thank God! Saturday, Tony went to Albany to help his sister Margaret and her husband with a roof repair. I'm so glad he could be in this part of the state so that he could help them. They have helped us so much. Hilary went to 5B for some red blood cells. During this process Hilary slept and I read. When we got home, Hilary slept for another four hours.

On Sunday, we watched two movies. For our outing, we drove to Safeway to pick up the Sunday paper. Then we sat in the car under a shade tree and read the paper. It was fun just getting out. Tony goes home Sunday evening. Today Tony picked more blackberries, so Hilary and I made some more pies. My job now is to look at those pies without eating myself sick. I'm gaining weight from eating foods that I fix for Hilary to gain weight. You'd think I would have more self-control.

Our lives are boring. It is wonderful. Thanks for your prayers. We have peace in a time that could be very stressful. That is God answering prayer.

Stay bored, everyone.

Love,

Jan

Chapter 5

SHAKING THE BOAT

Hilary update, Tuesday clinic
Tuesday, 13 August 2002

Well, today was *not* boring. We had an appointment with Dr. Fleming and we were told that the consensus of the doctors here at OHSU, and those they have called for conference across the U.S., is that Gabrielle is not a suitable donor for Hilary. Because they are identical twins, their stem cells are too similar for any graft advantage to happen. Also, too many of Hilary's chromosomes are abnormal. I asked what chromosomes were affected and Dr. Fleming said that the pathologist talked for three minutes explaining all the abnormalities. Apparently they looked at twenty chromosomes, and sixteen of them are not normal. Not good. Thus, Hilary absolutely needs a donor who will provide a graft versus leukemia[8] advantage, and Gabrielle's cells won't work out.

Yet the first order of business is to get Hilary into complete remission, which has not happened yet. We do another bone morrow test next Tuesday, and then we will know if the consolidation chemotherapy created remission. If not, Hilary will be given a different type of chemo to try to get this monster removed. Of course we are encouraging everyone to get themselves, their families, their friends, their neighbors, their work partners, their enemies (I'd even say their dogs, but I don't think they would qualify) on the national donor list. It would be one of the easiest ways to possibly save a person's life. Remind everyone of the chance to get on the list next Monday in Halfway for free. Call Dorothy for more information. Or, if you are close to Portland, you can do an apheresis on August 31 and move toward the list with only two more apheresis donations. Even if you can't do an apheresis, you can request your name to be added to the donor list. Anyway, that's how I think things work with the Red Cross.

During our devotion time this morning, I was very touched by the quote from Mark 6:50–51: "Take heart, it is I. Do not be afraid." Then Jesus got into the boat with the disciples. I knew that this was from the story of Jesus walking on the water and I wondered if Jesus' plan was to walk on by. Then when he saw the disciples afraid, he decided to get into the boat with them. So we read the whole story and, sure enough, that is what was indicated. Jesus climbs in our boat when we are afraid.

As the day progressed, I thought of how this day began. It is hard to hold Jesus' hand and feel his presence in the boat when it is shaking so hard. I know he is there; I just need to calm down. I'm waiting for the wind to stop blowing.

Talk to you later.

Love,

Jan

Donor Information

Hilary update
Thursday, 15 August 2002

I've had a few people ask for more information about the National Marrow Donor Program (NMDP). Here are a few facts:

- You must be between eighteen and fifty-five years old and in good health.
- You must donate a small sample of blood for tissue typing. There is a fee of around $100 to cover this blood test, but the Boise hospital and Red Cross are covering the fees at the Halfway blood drive on Monday.
- Your tissue type is entered into the NMDP's computerized registry. If the computer indicates you are a preliminary match for a patient, your donor center contacts you and, with your approval, you will need to donate another small sample of blood for more testing.
- After further testing, if you are a precise match for a patient, you will need to undergo a physical examination and, after being fully informed, you then decide whether to continue with the donor process.
- There are now two ways to donate stem cells. The old way was with a general anesthesia. The hospital does a simple surgical procedure to collect some bone marrow from your hip. Now, only a simple apheresis is needed to remove stem cells from your blood. Apheresis donors simply sit in a chair for a couple of hours as if donating blood. The blood is drawn from one arm and returned to the other arm after the stem cells are extracted.
- Your marrow and blood return to normal within a few weeks.

I'm sure you can look up more information on the internet, or call 1-800-MARROW-2.

According to one source, nearly 79 percent of patients needing new stem cells cannot find a suitable donor within their families and so they need to find an unrelated donor. The NMDP helps with that process.

I hope this helps.

Jan

Love, Jan

BLOOD DRIVE THANK YOU

Tuesday, 20 August 2002

Thank you, everyone, for all your support with the blood drive in Halfway. I've heard that it was extremely well-attended. Thank you, thank you, thank you. Maybe one of us will be chosen to help another person. Wouldn't that be wonderful! It would be just as exciting as winning the lottery.

Today we had clinic and Hilary had her day 28 bone marrow biopsy. We should know by Friday if she is in remission. I've had a few people ask what the bone marrow is matching when looking for a donor. They are looking for a human leukocyte antigen (HLA) match. These antigens are protein "markers" found on the surface of white blood cells.

When everyone started all the fundraisers, we felt it was unnecessary because we had excellent Blue Cross insurance with the 5J school district. Last week we found out Blue Cross doesn't cover a bone marrow search. Thus, we are especially grateful for all the fundraisers, because a bone marrow search can be very expensive. Kevin (our insurance agent) was very surprised, just as I was, that Blue Cross doesn't cover this part of our medical costs. How did you know that we would need this money? Thank you!

Last Wednesday I traveled back home to work in my classroom. Of course, everyone showered me with concerned comments. It makes me feel so loved. The administration even took time from their busy schedules to drive to Halfway to enter their blood in the donor bank. Only in Eastern Oregon would people drive 100 miles to help an employee. Isn't that wonderful!

I met my substitute. She will be covering for me on Fridays and during the transplant month. We had a great visit, and I think that we will be a good team for this class of third graders. They and I are lucky to have her.

Since Hilary's counts are high this week, she has us traveling to the beach today. Then on Thursday, we are going to the zoo. On Friday, Hilary enters the hospital for another five-day chemo treatment. Elizabeth and I head back to Baker County on Sunday. Thank you again for everything!

Love,
Jan

BEACH AND PLANE RIDE

Hilary update
Friday, 23 August 2002

Well, we are back at the hospital for Hilary's next chemo treatment. They are calling the results of the bone marrow biopsy from last Tuesday a bone marrow remission, but we won't know the results of the chromosomes until later. If they also show a remission, then we can celebrate! We will be one step closer to the transplant.

We had a great time visiting the beach. There is something renewing about the ocean. Grandma Bonn got to go with us, so we had an Irene with us (even if it wasn't the Irene we usually have). We stayed at my cousin Ron's beach house. Isn't that a wonderful gift? We don't want to overuse our welcome, but visiting the beach could be more often than the once-a-year event we are accustomed to.

We didn't get to visit the zoo on Thursday as planned. We'll try again during the next high-count week. Instead of the zoo visit, Brad Bonn (Hilary's cousin) took Gabrielle, Elizabeth, and Hilary for an airplane ride. They had a great time. This was Elizabeth's first time in a small plane. We joked about flying downtown where President Bush would be and seeing the action that would cause. They chose to fly south.

Gabrielle arrived very late Monday evening from Alaska. Hilary was very glad to see her! Even though Gabe was not going to be the

Love, Jan

transplant donor, she wanted to get here so she could spend some time with Hilary before college started. Maybe we'll have more time together as a family this year than I had anticipated.

I'd best close. Thanks again for the blood/donor drive. Thanks again for the medical funds you've given us. Thanks again for all the prayers. You are sooooo special! We are so privileged to know such wonderful people.

Love you,
Jan

COUNTING DAYS

Hilary update, day 60/day 2
Saturday, 24 August 2002

We are at day 2 of our next chemo treatment, but I'm counting day 60 from the time we entered OHSU. We convinced the doctors that we could do this treatment as an outpatient, so we only spent last night in the hospital.

This morning Hilary did her chemo in 5B, and then on the way back to the apartment, she and I went for a walk up a trail close to the hospital. Hilary is feeling cabin fever right now. We were hoping that a hike would help that problem. When we got to the apartment, Elizabeth and Gabrielle had left the following note:

Mom and Hilary,

We are currently walking to, or from, Safeway to cure the boredom that the naps ensued. We should be home shortly, depending upon when you happen to receive the pleasure of reading this brief, yet long-winded ramble of a note. Ha, ha.

Your daughters/sisters
Elizabeth & Gabrielle

They arrived just a few minutes after Tony. He did a short bow hunt with a friend of his brother Mike. He saw eight elk and came close to getting a shot at one. His comment is that "these elk are sure a lot bigger than those at home."

I'm already feeling the sadness of leaving, and I still have tonight to visit. Hilary told me, "Mom, you will be back on Thursday. That's not very long." For some reason, it feels like forever.

Hilary should be finished getting hooked up for her chemo treatment and a lady is waiting for the computer, so I'll say good-bye for tonight.

Love to you all.

> Prayerfully,
> Jan

PHYLLIS' STROKE

Hilary update, day 79/day 17
Sunday, 08 September 2002

I'm sorry I can't seem to get to the computer as often as I used to. So to all of you who write to me and I don't respond, please know that I promise to check my e-mail at least once a week.

An explanation of the day 79/day 17 at the top of the page: the first day is the entry day into OHSU, the last part of June. It is how long we have been fighting leukemia. Day 17 is the day of this consolidation. It keeps a record of where the blood counts should be.

Now the update information: Hilary was able to come back to the apartment yesterday. We are giving her the IV antibiotics here at the apartment. It is nice working with a home health group. The nurse comes to the home and explains everything, shows you how to do everything, and answers any questions. Very nice.

Yesterday, when the hospital nurse came to unhook the bag of platelets and said, "Well, you're free to go," Hilary literally jumped out of bed to put on her clothes. She was standing at the nurses' station desk while the nurse was hurrying to get the discharge papers in order. One nurse asked if they were that bad to work with. Hilary assured her that everyone was kind and helpful, but it was just time to go home. Hilary is (as always) feeling fine and has a great attitude. Her counts are starting to climb, so within about a week, she should be able to venture a little bit farther from the apartment.

For those of you who didn't know, Phyllis had a stroke last weekend. She is still in the hospital in Baker City. Dad, Melody, Erik, Amy, and Phil have been staying with her. Wade and Kathy have been checking on her daily. I'm concerned for Dad's stress levels.

Phyllis has lost complete use of her right side. She cannot talk. Her awareness is apparent, so she is working hard to help with her left side as much as possible. When she can sit for a three-hour period and is able to point, she will probably be moved to a rehab center. The hospital staff is working with communication skills and strength skills for that left side.

Because Dad is in Baker and Tony is in Portland, Chet C. is irrigating and caring for the ranch for us. Tony will be going to Richland this week, after Irene gets to Portland. Irene will be flying in tonight around 10:00. I am looking forward to seeing her next weekend! (I don't understand how people can handle crisis without family. What a team!)

Thanks for the prayers for my classroom and students. My Special Boy Number One was not defiant on day two of school (praise God); instead, he started harassing other students. On day three, he went home at noon, and Friday he did not come to school. He needs your continued prayers and I need prayer for wisdom, calmness, and continuity of discipline. He's lucky he is in my room, because he will have all your prayers for him.

Got to go if I'm going to make it to church. Love to you all.

Love,

Jan

COLLEGE AND SCHOOL

Hilary update
14 September 2002

Good morning, I am now at the apartment with Gabrielle while Irene and Hilary are at the hospital. Hilary re-entered the hospital last Monday because of a bacterial infection. We were treating one bacterium with Vancomycin, but Sunday evening her temperature returned. We still don't know what caused the new temperature. Hilary is hoping to return to the apartment by tomorrow. Her white count was one yesterday. When they become three, she can escape. She is certainly ready to do something different. I had her help me correct papers yesterday, which wasn't the something different she had in mind. We did get some great laughs while reading journals. Third-grade journals are precious.

Gabrielle registers for college in Klamath on the 26th. Thus, Tony is hoping to have everything in place on the ranch by that time so he can return to Portland. Irene is glad to be here in Portland, so she can help. She is busy making this apartment "her apartment" so she doesn't feel like a visitor. Irene has an interview for a job today, so of course I'm thinking about the schedule of Hilary sitters. Everything will work out.

Elizabeth is planning to move into her trailer apartment in La Grande, Oregon, this next week. She will be living with Brandi Wilson and Rebecca Bledsoe. I'm going to miss having her with me. She has been a rock for me all summer. More than once she has mentioned that if she were still at George Fox, she could help more in Portland. I know how she feels. I hope she likes Eastern Oregon University.

Phyllis is showing slight signs of progress. She will probably be in Baker for another week, and then some decisions will need to be made. Dad seems tired. I'm concerned about him.

My classroom is becoming settled. My Special Boy Number One, whom I've mentioned, is now living with his grandma and grandpa and is taking some medication for ADHD. He is better and I'm sure he will continue to improve. Thanks for your prayers.

Friday night I was able to stay with the Thompsons on the way down to Portland. It was great visiting with Tami (as always). Mike was on a trip with his job, so I missed seeing him. The kids are growing. Regina is taller than her mom. (I think they all will be taller than Tami.)

On my drive through The Gorge, the pink sunrise against the hills next to the Columbia River was absolutely gorgeous. I wish I could paint a picture with words. One truck driver was parked along the side of the road, walking around his truck and looking at the hills. It was well worth a stop!

I can't think of anything else interesting; besides, I need to prepare for a trip to the hospital. I love you all. Thanks for reading these reports and praying for us.

The "Car Queen,"
Jan

GLIDING

Hilary update
Saturday, 21 September 2002

Hello, everyone. Because Hilary's counts are high, we are having lots of fun. On Thursday the girls went to the zoo and to the Omnimax Theater. Friday, Irene signed some paperwork to work at The Reserve part-time. The Reserve is a restaurant at a members-only golf course. We ate there Friday night and it is really nice.

Today, Saturday, the girls were hurrying me out the door because they had a surprise for Hilary and me at Aunt Shelly and Uncle Mike's. When we drove out of the driveway, I informed Irene that she was going the wrong way, but she said, "We're going to be *with* Mike and Shelly, not *at* Mike and Shelly's."

We headed for the coast and I said, "Wow, the coast would be a great outing. I love going to the coast." Then we turned off of Highway 26 and I saw gliders. Brad, my nephew, pulls gliders almost every weekend, and today he was our guide in a glider. Hilary went first and had a great time. Then I got to go, and it was wonderful. I've always wanted to ride in a hot air balloon because I thought it would be quiet and I would be able to see the world. Well, the glider was quiet (a little wind sound) and I could see all the checkerboard farmland. It smelled so clean up there. Because of the wind, we had a few bumps, but that just made the ride better. We were pulled up by a yellow rope that looked just like the ropes used by water skiers. Brad even let us drop so we could feel the wake of the air from the tow plane. It reminded me of waterskiing until we let go and glided. From 4,000 feet up, everything is tiny, and you float and look right, float and look left, float and look up, float and wonder what is planted in that green field down there, float and relax. Fun!

Tony set all this up for us. Isn't that a wonderful surprise? I was sad that he couldn't be here to watch our faces. It is so wonderful to be so loved!

I love you and wish for you God's blessings. He is the best surprise-giver of all.

Love,

Jan

No Eyebrows

Hilary update

Sunday, 22 September 2002

I'm at school finishing a few things before I go to the hospital to see Phyllis. Phyllis is going to Boise tomorrow. Phyllis will be at the Elks Rehab. Of course, Dad is going with her to continue watching her therapy. While I was coming home today, I thought about how

Love, Jan

much I love Phyllis because I love my Dad. It made me think that there are people who love me because they know God, my Dad in Heaven. Interesting, isn't it?

Hilary has lost her eyebrows. She looks so different. I suggested an eyebrow pencil, but she doesn't care if she has eyebrows. She is still beautiful.

I've got to go.

I love you.
Jan

ROUTINES

Hilary update
25 September 2002

Hilary is sleeping through this week of chemo consolidation. Gabrielle is in Klamath Falls preparing for classes. Elizabeth will be in La Grande tomorrow preparing for classes. Irene is taking care of Hilary and working at The Reserve. Tony is looking into Portland Community College classes, but he will be in Richland for a few days caring for cattle. I am teaching school.

Hope everything is going well with you and your household. God bless.

Love,
Jan

MORE ROUTINES

Hilary update
Friday, 27 September 2002

I got to the hospital around 11:00 this morning. I stayed in Pendleton last night and left this morning around 8:00. The 360-mile drive to

Portland is always easy because I look for landmarks along the way. I like looking for elk in Ladd Canyon. I like thinking about the pioneers when I cross the Blue Mountains. I admire the poplar trees close to Boardman. I'm in awe of any wind surfers on the Columbia River. The landmarks going back to Baker on Sundays are not as interesting. Maybe it is because I have to leave part of my heart in Portland.

Hilary's last dose of chemo is tonight. She and Irene got to the apartment after this morning's treatment around 1:00 P.M. The first thing Hilary did was give me a hug. Then she went to bed. Chemo really makes her sleep! I told Irene that I would take Hilary for tonight's treatment and she could have some time to sleep, or clean. She has been either working or driving Hilary for treatments all week, and I know she would like some time to get some personal things finished. I'm glad I can be here to help.

I don't have a report on Phyllis. I tried to call Dad this morning and he didn't answer. I'll try again later.

Elizabeth's trailer house is still not ready. Now the plumbing is not working. She is more than frustrated. Her classes start on Monday, and I think she is planning on commuting for a few days if the trailer apartment is not ready. What a pain!

Gabrielle is getting settled, but her phone only calls out, so I can't call her. I'm so glad her Aunt Chris lives in Klamath. Chris is checking on Gabe and helping where she can. Family is so wonderful!

Irene has enjoyed her first week of work. Next week she is already scheduled for twenty-four hours. Maybe it will work into a full-time job.

Tony is helping Elizabeth move. He can tell the landlord about the problem with the plumbing, hook up the dryer, tell the landlord the problem with the stove, etc. I'm glad he is there for her. He plans on returning to Portland before Tuesday, when he has his classes to prepare for the nursing program. I can see his stress level rising as he tries to take care of all his girls.

I want to thank you for your prayers for my class. The field trip on Thursday was a great success. Two boys, Special Boy Number

Love, Jan

One and another friend, are testing my teaching skills. Both of them made it through the field trip with flying colors. Praise God. I've been sleeping less, trying to think of strategies for these boys. I was afraid that the lack of structure of a field trip could be disastrous. They made it! I was so excited! I am reminded again that I am not alone working with these kids. I have a partner, named Jesus, who is the master teacher!

Love to everyone,
Jan

RYAN

Hilary update
Sunday, 29 September 2002

I'm here at the school finishing up a few things before greeting students on Monday. Hilary finished her chemo consolidation Friday night at midnight. Saturday we rested. Her friend Ryan (a boy who entered the hospital the same time as Hilary, with the same disease, and only two years older than she) is not doing well. He contracted a fungus and the doctors told the family that the outcome depends on a rise in white blood cells. Things don't look good. He is in a lot of pain and delirious in the evenings. Hilary is concerned about him and realizes the importance of staying away from those microorganisms. She started this chemo with a low white cell count because of the infections she got last time her counts were low. I'm concerned. Seeing Ryan makes mortality real. We've had many discussions about cleaning the apartment and visiting friends. It is scary! Hilary's low counts start around Tuesday and will last for up to two weeks.

Please pray for Ryan. Got to go.

Love,
Jan

Germs

Hilary update
Sunday, 06 October 2002

Hilary is back in the hospital with a temperature. This has happened every single time her white counts get to zero. Friday evening, after I got to the apartment, I wasn't feeling normal. I didn't run a temperature, but I felt cold. I felt weak and not healthy. So, I stayed far away from Hilary and left Saturday by noon. I came back to La Grande and stayed with Elizabeth. (I was feeling sorry for her because she seems lonely. Her roommates don't have her same schedule and are not around much.) Then Hilary went into the hospital Saturday at midnight.

I am just going to have to stay home when her counts are low. I do work in the germ capital of the world called public school. This makes me feel horrible, that I may be the cause of this temperature. Tony assures me that the bacteria could come from anywhere, but he also agrees that I should stay home when Hilary's counts are low. I'm very sad! I'm praying that the antibiotics do the job and kill whatever is causing the temperature. Unfortunately, I keep thinking of Ryan and how bad he is because of these microorganisms. I need to remember that God is in charge and everything will be fine. Hilary belongs to the Creator and he takes care of His children!

Jan

Spot/Helgerson Fundraiser

Hilary update
Sunday, 13 October 2002

Hello, everyone. I have soooo much to say and it is already 8:00 P.M. You're going to get a slimmed-down version of everything.

Saturday the 5th: Hilary entered the hospital around midnight with a temperature.

Tuesday the 8th: The hospital staff took out her PICC line because after culturing her blood, they discovered that she had the same bacteria that she has fought every time her counts get low. They thought the PICC line might be the entry for the bacteria. (I wasn't to blame. Praise God.)

Thursday the 10th: They put in a new PICC line and in the process of x-ray they saw a spot on her lung. (Scary, worrisome spot. What could a spot mean?) They did a computerized axial tomography (CAT) scan. Then about midnight they started antifungal medicine in case the spot was a fungal infection.

Friday the 11th: They discussed what to do about the spot. They did an ultrasound of the heart, looking for bacteria around the heart valves. Decided to monitor and watch until today, when they will do another CAT scan to see if the spot is changing and how it is changing.

Saturday the 12th: I visited with the doctors about my staying with Hilary and they assured me that if I was free of any symptoms of illness. I could come, even if Hilary's counts were low. Yet, I shouldn't challenge my own immune system by getting close to ill people.

Helgerson/Portland Fundraiser:

Again we are so blessed! Irene kept saying that tears were brimming in her eyes. Elizabeth commented many times coming home about how much fun it was. It was *great*! I got to see some family and friends that I haven't seen for years. The music was absolutely awesome! The food was delicious! The auction gifts were beautiful and people seemed to have fun bidding. I know we made some money, but it isn't the money that makes the impression; it is the love of soooo many people. I thank each and every one of you for taking time from your busy lives to share with us your love. I know that some people were there because they loved someone who loves us. All those unknown people came to support someone else who loves us. Friends of the Helgersons came to support them, Peggy and Cal's friends came to support Peggy and Cal, some of my family came because they love my Dad, it is so far-extending. We were awestruck, honored, humbled, and blessed!

Thank you! Thank you! Thank you!

Jan

INTERNATIONAL SEARCH

Hilary update
Wednesday, 16 October 2002

They have started an international search for a donor. I'm praying that a perfect match shows up soon!

Hilary is still in the hospital. They took a sample of the spot in her lung yesterday. It will take a while to culture it so we know what we are fighting.

Phyllis will be moving back to Baker City within the next week. Progress is slow, but progress is happening. Thanks for the prayers.

I've got to correct a few papers and begin packing for Thursday's trip. Talk to you this weekend.

Love,

Jan

FUNGUS

Hilary update
Monday, 21 October 2002

Well, the nurse practitioner told Hilary yesterday (after I left) that the tests showed that the spot was a fungus. We don't know what treatment will follow besides the IV antifungal medicine that Hilary is receiving right now. Her counts are starting to climb, and she seems in good health, so this fungus isn't doing much right now. But we certainly need to be rid of it before she starts her last chemo treatment. The doctors seem to be in a big hurry to choose a donor and begin Hilary's transplant process. Tony is going to ask why they are in such a hurry. If Hilary is in remission, what is the hurry?

Hilary was released from the hospital on Friday night around 8:30. She was sooooooo excited. Two weeks of hospital was enough! Tom, Ly, and Louise visited Friday evening. Then Saturday, Hilary was in weekend clinic, receiving her antibiotics and antifungal medicines for five hours. We then drove through Washington Park before we got home. That evening Father Rob and Danielle G. visited. Sunday, we again went to weekend clinic, and I left for Richland when Hilary fell asleep. It's always hard leaving.

I'm really tired, so I'm going to close. Thank you again for all the prayers! I can feel your prayers; it is as if I am being carried. Hilary is a blessing to be around. No one is depressed when they are around Hilary. Peace and joy are certainly part of a situation that could be awful. It is God's hand carrying and comforting. There is no other explanation. Thank you for your prayers.

Love,
Jan

Ryan's Note

Hilary update
Saturday, 26 October 2002

This fall has been gorgeous! Fall has always been my favorite time of the year, but when fall began this year, I was disgusted and discouraged. I did not want it to be fall. However, fall seems to be doing its very best to be the most beautiful ever. During the last couple of weeks, I have truly enjoyed the colors and sun!

Patty and I had a big scare on our trip to Baker this last week. We came around a corner in the canyon and a cattle truck was in our lane. Of course, I pulled over onto the edge of the road. The truck was going around a bolder the size of my computer table. It was no one's fault, just two people hitting an unforeseen roadblock at the same time. The second truck stopped and was looking for a way to push the monster rock off the road. The third truck almost hit us, because he was crowding (really he was crossing the middle line) on a corner. He didn't expect to meet a car that early in the morning. Each time, Patty was saying her prayers, gripping the door, and complimenting me on my quick reflexes. I thought, "Isn't it strange, I drive to Portland every weekend and my most dangerous driving is twenty miles from my home."

I debated for a week about coming to Portland this weekend. I developed a cough. The cough didn't arrive with a sore throat or runny nose. It just showed up. I had Hilary ask her doctors about it, and they said, "As long as the cough was allergy-related I didn't need to worry about not visiting." So, then I worry, is this allergy-related? Is it worth taking a chance? I'm here, keeping my distance.

Hilary is taking the antifungal medicine as an outpatient. So the apartment has a hospital pole with a pump for the four-and-a-half-hour infusion. Aunt Mary said Jerome called this medicine "shake and bake." It is truly a great description! After the infusion last night, Hilary's teeth chattered while I was heating blankets in the oven to pile over the blankets already surrounding her. Then within a half hour, she acted like a hot-flash victim and was down to a T-shirt. I knew this medicine was strong stuff when last weekend the nurses gave Hilary an EKG after the treatment at weekend clinic. Living in Eastern Oregon, I couldn't understand why the doctors wanted to do a surgery to remove this fungus. Surgery sounds so invasive. Now, I hope they do the surgery next week, so Hilary doesn't have to take this awful medicine much longer.

All of Hilary's counts are coming up, but the white counts are dropping just a little. I think it is because of the fungal fight. I've also wondered why the doctors seem to be in such a hurry to find a donor, since Hilary seems to be doing so well. I can now see how her body is weakening. This fungal fight is not easy, so I'm beginning to understand the urgency in finding a donor.

Tony and Hilary told me that Ryan went home to die. Ryan and his family were headed for the coast yesterday. He refused a different treatment for the leukemia that seemed to never leave. He still has his liver fungus, and then another bacteria decided to live with him. He and his girlfriend sent Hilary a card through the nurses. It had four 12-inch watercolor white cells with a note saying, "Ryan and I wanted you to have these white blood cells to help you recover and be well. Thank you for being so special and loving." I hope and pray that peace envelopes them and that they let Jesus shepherd them.

Death is not an ending; it is just a temporary separation. Yet, thinking about that temporary separation makes me cry.

Dad and Phyllis are in Baker again. They don't know how long they will be allowed to stay at the hospital. Improvement seems to be the key word. Phyllis' improvement doesn't seem to be substantial enough to please the hospital staff. I got to watch the speech therapist work with Phyllis, who seems to be trying hard. Dad has a lot of decisions he needs to make. Melody, Phyllis' daughter, should be there today, and maybe they together can make a plan.

Gabrielle loves Klamath Falls. She gets along great with her roommate. Elizabeth is adding activities to her schedule. Irene just bought a couch, loveseat, chair, and ottoman, so Tony is starting to return some of this wonderful loaned furniture.

I thought of Pine Eagle and homecoming. I hope the football and volleyball games went in our favor. Sarah's volleyball team is playing in the playoffs at Hermiston on Monday. I wish I could go and watch. Keep us posted on events in your lives. We enjoy hearing from you! Seize each day! And love the Creator, who gave it to you.

Love,
Jan

FINDING CORD BLOOD

Hilary update
Tuesday, 29 October 2002

Tony called me at school today and said they found a cord blood out of Germany that only mismatches in one spot. It will work. I felt a weight lift (I didn't know I was carrying it). Then I did a dance! (Celebration for the soul.) I'm now praying that the graft versus host (GVH) problem will not be too large a cross to carry. Before a transplant can take place, the fungus needs to be gone. So as I learn more about the fungal fight, I'll let you know.

I asked Hilary if she was excited about finding a donor and she said that she was not surprised. They have been saying for a couple of weeks that if nothing better shows up, that this cord blood will work. I think her thoughts are that it might be second best to something they can't find. I come back to the thought that Jesus came second;, God was first but when we couldn't get things right, Jesus came. It is Jesus who saves, heals, and gives us life. Second place is just right!

Love,
Jan

CORD BLOOD

Hilary update
Friday, 1 November 2002

I've had a few people ask questions about donor cord blood. Here is a little information:

HLA typing, which maps the protein markers found on white cells, determines a donor match. The hospital looks at six markers, which are inherited through the genes passed down from the parents—three from the mother and three from the father. There are two A antigens, two B antigens, and two DR antigens. Hilary is mismatched on one DR with this cord blood.

A cord blood is an umbilical cord. The umbilical cord is drained of blood and the blood is taken to a cord blood bank and frozen. Approximately three to five ounces of blood can be collected. Hilary can use a cord blood because she weighs less than 110 pounds. Umbilical-cord blood doesn't require as close an HLA match as an adult donor.

This cord blood is from Germany and they sent over a small sample to OHSU for further testing. It was this further testing that gave the doctors confidence that this cord blood will be a good donor for Hilary.

The fungal fight is in wait mode until Hilary's white cell count gets to three. Wednesday, her counts were at 1.4. I've seen white cell counts jump fairly quickly, but I've also seen them creep along. We'll wait. And while we wait, we will seize each day and thank God for all his blessings! You are one of those many blessings. Thank you again for all your prayers.

Love,

Jan

Chapter 6

Hilary update
Friday, 08 November 2002

This week has turned us around again. I will start with Tuesday's clinic.

Hilary started the day with a CAT scan to check the fungus size. Then when she visited with the doctors, she was informed that they saw a few abnormal cells from Friday's bone marrow test. Even though her white cell count was high enough for surgery, her platelet count was not.

Wednesday, I cried all the way to Baker. I was glad I had a classroom of students with their own problems to take my mind off of my thoughts. Wednesday night I came to La Grande to watch Elizabeth's symphony concert. Tony came to do some work on the ranch, so we met in La Grande and had a nice evening together.

Thursday, Tony called me around 3:00 to say there was a message from Irene. The leukemia was back. He told me about the plan of attack, but I couldn't focus much. After conferences, I called Hilary. The leukemia was back and Gabrielle was coming to the rescue. The problem was how to treat the returned leukemia with chemo (which would allow the fungus to take control of the body) or whether to continue fighting the fungus with the slow medicine attack (which would allow the leukemia to take control of the body). They plan to use Gabrielle's identical twin stem cells (do a transplant) to control the leukemia. Then when Hilary's white cells are gone, they will apheresis Gabe for white cells to fight the fungus. Gabrielle is talking to her professors today about a three-week absence from school. She will be in Portland by Sunday, and we have a meeting with Dr. Fleming on Monday morning.

To use the cord blood now would require a larger chemo attack, and the fungus would yell, "My turn, my turn." We have to fight both and win both battles at the same time.

I want you to know that Hilary's first words to me were, "Don't worry! Mom, this will work. But if it doesn't, we are all going to die someday, anyway. If this leukemia takes me, worrying doesn't change anything. This is going to work, anyway. I'm just very lucky that I have an identical sister; otherwise the story might be different."

She is very positive, and angry with anyone who shows her that worried look. She is confident of the fight! She talks of death and doesn't seem afraid. It's out there someday, and nothing will stop it. Worrying doesn't change anything but how we live and enjoy today. Don't worry!

The amazing thing about these words is that Hilary truly means them. She is not just talking. She seems truly at peace with her situation, with the fight she is waging. She is a stronghold and comfort for all the rest of us. I have never heard her say, "Why me?" Paul talks about "the peace that passes all understanding." I'm seeing this in Hilary. This has to be Jesus. I know of no other way to receive this kind of peace.

Talk to you later.

Love,
Jan

CENTRAL LINE

Hilary update
Saturday, 16 November 2002

Sorry I haven't written sooner. This is the first time I've made it to a computer to check my e-mail. I'm trying to get organized, which is a major undertaking for me. If you want proof of my scattered mind, just take one look at my desk. Hilary entered the hospital on Wednesday. She took some anti-seizure medicine in preparation for the chemo she started on Thursday.

Thursday they put in a central line. So she now has a PICC line and a central line. The central line starts at the middle of the chest. It goes under the skin until it reaches the collarbone. At the collarbone, the line enters the jugular vein and travels to the heart. Right now, this central line is very sore in one spot and itches in another. She started her chemo on Thursday. The chemo comes in the form of pills instead of an IV infusion, and if she takes those capsules too fast they don't stay in her stomach. Last night when I got here, she seemed exhausted but didn't want us to leave until 10:00 P.M., when she was due to take her pills.

Grandpa came with us, and Hilary was very glad to see him. August was the last time he was able to visit. Elizabeth came with him and they will head home on Sunday, but I get to stay here. The whole floor staff said, "We wondered where you were. It's about time you got here." Because we lived on floor 5C for a month, when Hilary first came from Alaska, it feels like Old Home Week. When Hilary needed to stay in the hospital for bacterial infections, she stayed on 5A. She likes 5C a whole lot better; it is more like a family.

When we got here this morning, Hilary was sleeping. (Gabrielle is staying with Hilary at the hospital.) She didn't get much sleep the night before. Apparently around 1:00 A.M. she started running a temperature, so they took an x-ray and started her on antibiotics. Of course, I start worrying that I may have brought her a third-grade bug. They are doing blood cultures to find out all about the little visitor. Maybe it is the sore central line, maybe it is too many visitors, and maybe it is her hot room. (Irene likes the room to stay around eighty degrees. I'm cooking but when I turn down the heat, Hilary gets cold. I'll cook. When I mentioned the hot room to the nurse at the nurse's station, they just smiled and said they leave waving their arms. It reminds me of my room at school, but I can't open the window.)

Well, I'll write more later. Stay cool.

Love to all,
Jan

Three Days until Transplant

Hilary update
Monday, 18 November 2002

Hilary is sleeping right now. She is finished with the buphosiphine (sp) and today she takes a four-hour infusion of a different chemo. Then she gets two days off before transplant. Gabrielle is over at clinic, getting her Neupogen shot (Neupogen causes the body to increase stem cells) and taking a chemistry test. Her professor faxes the test to the clinic social worker. When Gabe is finished taking the test, Nancy, the social worker, faxes it back. I think it's great that the clinic and BMT team are helping Gabrielle work with Oregon Institute of Technology (OIT) to finish her classes. I'm praying that she does well! It is hard to do classes over e-mail and by just reading the book. There is a purpose to going to class and listening to an expert on a subject.

Elizabeth told me that I needed to do something besides sit in a hospital room and hover over Hilary, so I decided I would go to daily Mass. I thought of Walt Parker. One of his heart's desires is to attend daily Mass, and now I have an opportunity to take advantage of that service. During Sunday Mass I always cry. I thought I was going to make it through an entire service yesterday without tears, but then the words "joyful hope in Christ Jesus" just rang and rang and rang inside my head and I started to cry. Poor Tony, having to put up with me wiping my eyes.

Today I prayed on my walk to church that Jesus would show through me. That the "joyful hope" could shine forth. After Mass the lady next to me asked my name and told me that I just glowed. I told her that it must be Jesus, and she said, "Thank you, I needed to see Jesus today." Wow! If Jesus answers such a simple prayer, I know he will answer my constant prayers. Besides, I felt the best part of Mass today were the prayers of the faithful. Many prayers were said by those older saints who are able to attend daily Mass. I hope they know how powerful and needed they are. I am learning over and over again about how powerful prayer is. We are not alone or weak when we have Jesus as a partner. Thank you for your prayers, and we want you to know that we pray for you each day too.

Joyfully hopeful in Christ Jesus,

Jan

HILARY, DAY - 2

Hilary update
Tuesday, 19 November 2002

Yesterday afternoon was a carefully watched chemo. I don't remember its name, but apparently everyone who has a transplant gets it. When the nurse told us that she would be taking Hilary's vitals every fifteen minutes during the four-hour infusion, I knew this one was different. They put a blood pressure machine on her so they could check blood pressure easily (and look at the heartbeat, etc.). Hilary's blood pressure did drop, and then later during the night her blood pressure dropped to 73 over 35 which is pretty low, so all night they continued checking the pressures. Today she was *very* tired.

I'm glad that poison is done! Now she has two days' rest before the transplant on Thursday.

Gabrielle's only side effects for her shots are horrible headaches. I've told people that donating stems cells is easy, but maybe it isn't. One little gal down the way ended up in the emergency room because she reacted to the pain medication they gave her for her bone pain. I'm glad Gabe's bone pain is just in her head and not in her whole body. Donating stems cells or bone marrow is still a wonderful possibility for saving a life. I think it would be awesome to be chosen to help someone.

Irene has strung Christmas lights all around Hilary's room. Whenever someone enters, they comment on how cozy the room is. We've had more than one hospital employee mention how wonderful our daughters are. One patient who was being released told Kelly, one of the nurses, "You take care of that Hilary."

Hilary's hair and eyebrows are growing back. They make Hilary extra beautiful. Her hair is so soft that it feels like the nose of a horse. I love to rub her head, and she loves to have her head rubbed. Good combination. I need to go.

> Prayerfully,
> Jan

HILARY, DAY –1

Hilary update
Wednesday, 20 November 2002

Today was a very nice day—the last day Hilary could leave the floor. So before imprisonment, we took a walk on the sky bridge, visited Mike Fash [sp] from New Bridge, and sat in the lobby while listening to a woodwind quintet (the hospital was celebrating being selected as Oregon's first provider, so they were serving punch and cake).

Gabrielle was fighting a headache again today, but that is normal. She needs to be on the floor for apheresis by 7:30 tomorrow morning. I'm guessing the transplant will be finished by noon. The doctors still say that we are only doing this transplant because of the situation Hilary is in right now. They still want to do a transplant with the cord blood just as soon as Hilary is well enough to start treatment again. I'm praying that Gabe's stem cells will give Hilary a little GVH problem so that this will be it. That would be a miracle. God knows the plan. He is in control, but in my mind it would be a very nice solution. Of course, I've always been a person who would take the easy way out if I could. There is no harm in asking. God can say yes, or he can say no. We'll see. Wouldn't that surprise the doctors?

Got to go. I'll talk to you tomorrow.

Love,
Jan

Transplant Day

Hilary update, day 0
Friday, 22 November 2002

Yesterday was an uneventful day for a day that should carry lots of enthusiasm. Those life-giving cells don't make any noise when they move from place to place. There are no bows or "Here we are!" shouts. They just march, or rather slowly flow, right in and go to work.

Tony and I arrived at the hospital around 7:20 and escorted Gabrielle to the apheresis room. They asked Gabe if she had eaten breakfast, which of course she hadn't because she didn't get up until 7:10 A.M. You know how college kids' schedules work. Consequently, the first order of the day was to take Gabrielle down to the diner for an omelet, potatoes, and very little water.

Around 9:00, she was settled, unable to bend either arm because each arm had an IV attached to it. Those arms were part of a circuit to remove and return her blood. When the blood is out of the body, a machine apheresis or spins the stem cells away. My job was to scratch the nose, move the hair, rub the feet, and read her next lesson in the psychology book. I read three pages and she fell asleep. No excitement in psychology.

While we were there, we met some very sick people. One lady on oxygen, with a skin color of grayish green, came in for a transfusion because of a disease that affects her hematocrits. The room was dancing because they were able to get into her veins and do the transfusion. It has been two years since the last process. She was looking forward to getting off oxygen. She wanted to be able to care for her four little girls better.

Then a boy about nine years old came in. This visit for apheresis was "old hat" for him. He talked about seeing the latest Harry Potter movie and about having lost ten pounds (fluids) after the last treatment. Cute kid, and he talked with those nurses as if he were twenty, not nine, years old. I think being sick causes children to either become mature beyond their years or more childish than their years. They don't act their age.

At noon, Gabe was finished, and the first place to visit was the bathroom.

We headed back to 5C, and Hilary was ordering a yogurt shake because she didn't fill out the menu the day before and didn't like what the kitchen had sent up. At 1:00 P.M., the entire bone marrow transplant (BMT) staff and clinic had a Thanksgiving dinner on the floor for everyone, including patients and families. Hilary ate a little turkey and ham. The rest of us ate until we were uncomfortable. While I was eating, I met a lady who was a donor for her sister, and she (with her husband) are missionaries in Austria. Wow! Then to make the story better, one of the churches that supports their work is the Baptist Church in Halfway, Oregon. They have been to Halfway and know some of the people there. I remember Laurie asking me if we had met a Barbara yet. Well, we have now. Isn't it a small world!

Midway through the afternoon Ralph came around to take some pictures. I had asked Debbie if she knew of anyone with a digital camera so that I could e-mail pictures. Brother Ralph was so nice to take time to do the honors. Hopefully you got a copy of them. I think they are wonderful.

Then Dr. Blizzard, the fungi surgeon, came to visit. Hilary introduced me and I kept thinking this guy reminds me of Chris. When I mentioned it to Wade and Kathy over the phone, Irene very quickly said, "It was the shape of his face and his blue, blue eyes." I was glad someone else noticed.

Dr. Blizzard is still on call for a surgery we might have yet to do. If there is scar tissue from the fungi, then they will do surgery to remove the scar tissue because some dormant cells might be hiding in it.

About 2:00, the stem cells arrived for Hilary. The nurse took vitals, blood pressure, and temperature, etc., every five minutes during the two-hour infusion. Hilary slept or tried to sleep with an interruption every five minutes for vitals. We all sat, read, watched, and slept a little throughout the infusion. Very boring! Isn't that wonderful?!

Around 6:00, they told us the count of stem cells Gabe gave to Hilary. If there were not enough, Gabe would have had to do apheresis again today, and Hilary would have received another batch. Some hospitals only require 2 million cells for a transplant. OHSU requires 5 million cells. Gabrielle gave Hilary 12 million cells. The nurses were so surprised at the amount. Gabe, of course, just flexed her muscles and smiled.

Todd arrived around 5:00. He and Gabrielle went to the movies. Today we are celebrating the girls' nineteenth birthday. The hospital is calling today Hilary's second birthday, because yesterday was a birthday too. It was a stem cell new birth.

Tony and I got home around 11:00 P.M. We waited for Gabrielle to get back from the movies. Irene had gone over to Nicky's to work on plans for a birthday party. Who knows what everyone is doing. I'm just

Love, Jan

showing up. I'm terrible at party things. (I'm wrapping Irene's gifts and supporting everyone's ideas.)

Thank you for all your prayers. We live one day at a time and today we celebrate birthdays. Please celebrate something today. I do believe God wants us to be joyful. We have a "joyful hope" in Christ Jesus. Isn't that wonderful? What a promise!

Love,
Jan

HILARY, DAY 3

Hilary update, day 3
Tuesday, 26 November 2002

It is Sunday morning around 11:00. I'm going to write a little and save the draft. It took me half an hour to get this hospital computer to open Hotmail and I have laundry ready to go from the washer to the dryer. The hospital has a washing machine and dryer, plus a shower, for family members who are staying with patients. Unfortunately, the dryer takes ninety minutes to dry a small load of clothes. I'm glad Hilary chooses to wear her cute pajamas instead of hospital gowns. I don't mind doing laundry. It puts some normal tasks into an abnormal life.

4:00 P.M.: the girls are listening to *Harry Potter*. It was so nice of Ann to loan the books to us. Irene says she's hooked! Hilary has read all the books and can't wait for book five, but Irene has not read any of them. Hilary wanted Irene to read them, and listening to them is fun for all of us.

Including *Harry Potter*, Hilary and I are involved in three different books. We're almost finished with *Sweetness to the Soul* by Jane Kirkpatrick. It was recommended by Kay and Harland at the fundraiser. We can only read it when Gabrielle is around because she, too, is enjoying hearing it. A week after Kay recommended the book, the author came

78

to Baker for a high tea, with the proceeds being given to the 5J school district library fund. Isn't it coincidental that Kay mentions this book and the author visits Baker within such a short time? So I went to Betty's Books in Baker City and cashed in my gift certificate from Churchill. It's been fun reading about The Dalles area. The last book we are reading is an unpublished book by a cancer survivor given to us by Judith Allan. This author lives here in Portland and her book, *Out of the Lines*, will be on the shelves soon.

We do a lot more reading than watching TV to pass the time. It is fun being able to stop and discuss something.

Now a quick review of the birthday celebration: Irene and Todd made a spicy bean soup, while I wrote e-mails and wrapped gifts. When we got to the hospital, Hilary had just finished with a nausea problem (it seems to happen daily). She didn't want to embarrass any friends, so we kept the day to family, staff, and patients on 5C. We had a lot of soup left over. After soup and opening gifts, Judith gave Hilary a craniosacral therapy treatment. These treatments seem to give Hilary energy, and she loves them. The hospital is supportive of the treatments. Judith is a chiropractor and doesn't promote craniosacral therapy as a main part of her practice, but it is growing by word of mouth. I'm sure Hilary will probably really promote this with her massage business when all of this is over. Later that day, Teisha came by and sang a couple of songs. It was wonderful! While Teisha was here, Father Jim from St. Elizabeth's Church came by, singing "Happy Birthday" to the tune of the "Hallelujah Chorus." He said he tried three times to get in to see us. I'm glad he was persistent. The girls received some beautiful cards, scarves, T-shirts, candy, candles, a dart game, a paint set for Hilary, and some sun glasses for Gabe. It was another day filled with love, and it was fun just being together.

Today Hilary's counts are .6 and Gabe is taking her Neupogen shot around 6:00 P.M., so she can do apheresis tomorrow morning for Hilary's white cell infusion. I asked Hilary if she could feel the fungus, but she can't. Isn't it a miracle that our body just quietly fights these invisible intruders and we don't even know it? We aren't even aware of the battle within our own bodies. I asked Hilary if she thought her body's fighting defenses had abandoned her. She told me that she thought her body was working very hard, but it just got overtaken. That's when outside reinforcements need to come and help. That is so true for all ailments. This reminds me of the reading today where Matthew talks about us being separated from God because we didn't feed the hungry, visit those in prison, give water to those in need. We need to be the reinforcements in life. I feel those reinforcements in my life. Hopefully I can be that for other people.

Monday, 10:30 P.M.

Just as I was finishing this, Irene came down and told me that the staff found vancomycin-resistant enterococci (VRE) in Hilary's stool. VRE is a bacterium that does not respond to the antibiotic vancomycin. The protocol for keeping it contained is to isolate Hilary in her room. We family members need to wash our hands as we leave the room, as well as before we enter the room, and we cannot touch anything when we leave. So, we are now banned from the computer, microwave, water jug, etc. All staff members need to be gowned and gloved when they enter the room. (At least we family members don't have to wear gowns all day.) I, of course, started asking questions because this sounded serious! All of the precautions are for the other patients. Hilary has the bacteria, but the bacterium is not active within her and so she is not sick. Since these particular bacteria can stay dormant on clothing and surfaces for up to three weeks, we can't touch anything. We are just trying to protect the other patients on floor 5C. I've noticed that four doors out of nine have the same isolation poster on their door, so I think the bacteria is moving no matter the precautions. Anyway, I'm now at the apartment and trying to finish this long e-mail. I think I'll save a draft again because I'm tired.

Tuesday morning, 9:30 A.M.

I need to leave for the hospital. I slept in and I'm running late. I promised Gabrielle that I'd be early (ha, ha) so she could go take a math test at the clinic. Judith is coming this morning. I'm hoping Hilary is feeling better. Yesterday she really fought nausea and I heard her cough a couple of times (my signal that the fungus is growing again). I'll probably miss seeing the doctor, which I don't like. I need to hurry, but I wanted to get this sent. You'll probably not get another e-mail for a while because we can't use the computer at the hospital and I'm not at the apartment much. Love you all.

P.S. Phyllis is doing very well, according to Dad. She is home with some outside help. They are getting into a routine and she is continuing to improve. Thank you, God! Also, some people have asked about my girls after seeing the pictures. Elizabeth was not here in Portland the day of the stem cell transplant, so she is not in the photos. I feel bad that we took pictures without her, because she is so very important to us and a very important part of our lives. She wishes daily that she could be here and not in La Grande. It is harder on people who are away than on those of us who are here. I think of the war wives who had to stay home when their husbands were across the sea. Of course this comparison is weak, because we are not at war (or are we?). Oh bother, I need to go. I love you.

THANKSGIVING

Hilary update
Thursday, 28 November 2002

I came to the apartment with Gabrielle to help put away the food and thought I'd check the e-mail. It is so much fun reading your notes.

I'm not going to be Rambling Rod today, just going to give a fast update. Hilary doesn't seem to mind her isolation, but she is not exercising. I'm talking to the staff about putting a sheet on the bike and letting Hilary wear gloves. So far the infection expert has not OK'd the bike plan. I think I'm more bugged about not being able to use the conference room than Hilary is about the bike. Oh, well.

Hilary is starting to get a few mouth sores. She grimaces every time she tries to swallow. Just remember a horrible sore throat and you will know what she is fighting. I don't think it is as bad as Mark or Yvonne's mouth sores. Probably Gabe's white cells are helping Hilary. Hilary's white count today was .7. Whenever I hear her cough, I thank God that Gabrielle is such a willing blood bank.

Irene fixed a wonderful Thanksgiving dinner. We all ate in the hospital room, and one staff member mentioned to Hilary about how lucky she was to have such a wonderful family. I am thankful for my family.

We received the video of the "Over the Hill For Hilary" walk. Thanks, Stephanie! We've watched it three times.

We received the book called *When Cancer Meets God*. Thanks Rachel! After we read it, we are going to leave it on the floor for other patients. Because of this book, I reread the story about David and Goliath. Did you know that David said, "The battle belongs to the Lord," before he went in to fight Goliath? We trust while we are moving. We don't sit back and wait.

Got to go, or everyone will think we had a wreck getting to the apartment.

Love to you all.

I hope you had a Thankful Thanksgiving.

Love,

Jan

Mouth Sores

Hilary update, day 9, Saturday
Saturday, 30 November 2002

After my shower, I decided to get on the computer in the conference room before I reentered Hilary's isolation room. This computer truly taxes a person! After a half hour I was going to give it one more try, and it must have known it was time to stop teasing me. *Ohhhhhhhhh!*

Quick update: Hilary lost her hair again on Thursday evening. She didn't want to lose it again but said, "I know it will grow back." The mouth sores are absolutely awful! She now has a suction tube (like you have at the dentist) which is so much better than using up a box of Kleenex every four hours. The throat is simply too painful to swallow. One nurse explained that high-dose chemo and radiation cause the lining of the gut (mouth and anus) to slough off. The lining is destroyed and only grows back with engraftment. This dying tissue is very, very painful. So painful, in fact, a person doesn't even want to swallow their own saliva. Hilary looks forward to her showers and Judith's craniosacral massages. Other than that, this vacation needs to be finished. Hilary is ready to move on to something different.

Gabrielle's arms are tired and sore. What a strong gal. It took them three tries yesterday to find two veins that would cooperate. They finally went into the same arm in two different spots. At least Gabe had a free arm to bend. She never complains. I think they are going to let her go back to Klamath Falls.

Elizabeth plans to leave today and go to Richland to visit Grandpa and Phyllis. This mother hen likes to have everyone around, but I know that the chicks need to move on with their lives. I'm glad I get to stay with my bald-headed gal!

Talk to you later when I'm at the apartment on a friendlier computer. This computer doesn't like me!

Love,
Jan

Love, Jan

DAY 9, SATURDAY AND NOW SUNDAY

Hilary update, day 9
Sunday, 01 December 2002

Yesterday was more of the same, with awful mouth sores. Hilary is now taking morphine to cut the pain. This is surely the worst part. I'm planning to drive Gabrielle back to Klamath Falls today. Her job of sharing stem cells and white cells is finished. She is hoping she is not too far behind in her classes at OIT. Irene will stay with Hilary, and Tony is doing some research for a paper he needs to write for school. Hilary's plan is to grow some white cells to fight the mouth sores. We are anxious for engraftment of Gabe's stem cells into Hilary's bone marrow, where Hilary marrow will produce those fighting white cells.

ENGRAFTMENT

Hilary update, day 11
Tuesday, 03 December 2002

Good news: Hilary's white cells are coming in. The engraftment is taking hold.

Bad news: Hilary's temperature went to 104. They are doing some tests (blood cultures, CAT scan, etc.) but she can't keep anything in her stomach, so Tylenol doesn't stay down. She has ice packs under her arms and cold cloths on her head. She is really sick!

I took Gabe to Klamath Falls and as I moved through the fog around Medford and Grants Pass, I thought about how time is unknown in the fog. You can't tell where the sun is and so time doesn't seem right. It is also hard to move forward in the fog without road signs and maps. As I'm straining my eyes to see the next curve that I don't want to miss for fear of a wreck, the scripture from the first part of Isaiah 40:4 (TEV)

84

"Fill every valley; level every mountain." It could say to straighten every curve and give light in the fog.

Wednesday update: Hilary's counts today were 10. This is a huge increase from yesterday. The doctors say the mouth, throat, and GI tract sores should be finished within a couple of days. The nausea is an individual fight, and so we wait.

The CAT scan showed a disappearing fungus. I don't think surgery will be needed. Thank God!

After a 105 temperature yesterday, the staff used a Tylenol suppository. Usually suppositories are not used on 5C because of low platelet counts. Today the temperature didn't get above 103. We still have no reason for the high temperatures, but the theory is an overworking immune system. Gabe's stem cells went in and said, "Hey, what is going on in here? This place is a mess." Then in their flurry to clean up, the body is getting very warm. I'm praying that it is engraftment that is causing the temperature.

Love,

Jan

CRANIOSACRAL THERAPY

Hilary update, day 15
Friday, 06 December 2002

Good morning, everyone,

I'm here at the apartment after an uninterrupted night's sleep. I've been staying at the hospital most nights, but Irene stayed last night because she is working the next two days (we fight over who gets to stay with Hilary).

Yesterday they started Hilary on total parenteral nutrition (TPN), which is liquid food. Really it is vitamins and sugars in a bag. They didn't want to start them because it means that Hilary will be in the hospital for at least another five days. She gets a finger prick four times a day to make sure the blood sugar doesn't go bonkers. Plus, they really watch the liver function. The nausea just isn't any better. Yesterday she ate two bites of yogurt, two bites of hamburger, and two bites of Jell-O. Nothing stayed down. I'm glad they put her on the liquid food. She took one short walk down the 5C hall (of course, after putting on a gown and gloves) and her legs were a bit shaky. As we said the Lord's Prayer yesterday, I was praying that the food would stay down and strength would return when we said, "Give us this day our daily bread."

Just a little information about craniosacral, for those of you who have asked: Dr. John Upledger noticed the pulsation of the spinal cord during a brain surgery when he was a student. When he asked about it, he was told that the pulsation was always there, but his instructors did not have much more information. He has since studied and evaluated the function of the membranes and fluid that protect the brain and spinal cord. Craniosacral therapy (CST) enhances those functions. He claims that it is not an alternative medicine, but a complementary, integrative, avant-garde area of medicine. He just testified before the House of Representatives about the responsiveness of autism to CST. And the latest study is showing that CST can relieve posttraumatic stress disorder in Vietnam vets who have suffered for twenty to thirty years. If you want more information, look at www.craniosacraltherapy. com.

I know that Hilary is stronger for at least twelve hours after a therapy session. The hospital doesn't frown on her sessions. Hilary says she hopes she gets craniosacral training in her massage classes.

Here are some interesting statements:

When God and Cancer Meet, by Lyn Eib: "Worrying about tomorrow robs today of its job."[9]

I think the holocaust survivor Corrie Ten Boom said the following: Life is 10 percent what happens to us and 90 percent how we respond to it.

SKY BRIDGE CAROLERS

Hilary update, day 18
Monday, 09 December 2002

Good morning, everyone.

Hilary usually sleeps until noon, so I came to the apartment to help Tony type his school paper and check e-mail. It is always so nice to hear from everyone.

Hilary has certainly turned the corner in healing. She has not vomited since Friday. I thought a couple of times she was going to lose it, but she held on and everything stayed down. Saturday morning, Kristin, Hilary's nurse, asked if maybe I could get the pills into Hilary with ice cream. Hilary had not taken pills for five days, and the liver pill seemed to be an important medicine to get down. Throughout the week Hilary tried many suggestions on how to get the medicine to go down. She tried chocolate ice cream. She tried pudding. I asked her if it was the throat or the stomach that was rejecting this important pill. She said "the pill" was in constant down/up motion and she couldn't tell where the body was yelling, "No way, Jose." I asked the doctors if we could we place this famous pill as a suppository (a suggestion of Nancy's), but they said this pill needed the stomach acids to help the digestion and absorption. So on Saturday we tried vanilla ice cream. I didn't know if taking the pill was becoming a psychological roadblock or if the pill was the true problem.

Because Hilary was sleeping, I hid "the pill" into a bite of ice cream and told her to just swallow. She gagged a little, but it went down. She said, "There was a pill in there. You are lucky I didn't bite down." I told her to go back to sleep and if the pill stayed for ten minutes, we'd try the rest of her pills then. It worked! It was the beginning of a wonderful day. She finished the day with 660 calories and 11 oz. of fluid. Not much for a healing body, but Saturday was a great beginning.

My job now is suggesting different foods or drinks. Irene made some almond milk, but that didn't work. Tony's fried venison was a hit. Hilary's throat is still very sore and so swallowing is still a job, but a job she is doing. Her tongue is smooth after all the scabs have left. She has no taste buds, so food isn't fun; it is a job. Of course, I had just read about Daniel, Shadrach, Meshach, and Abednego and how they didn't want to defile themselves with the food from the king. Here I eat anything I want, knowing that sugar isn't good for my body. We all have trouble with this business of eating. Self-control is my battle. As I watch Hilary fight to get things down, I admonish myself to stay true to my battle with eating too much sugar.

We finished reading *Outside the Lines* by Annette Mattern. It was good for Hilary to hear about a cancer survivor's fight with nausea. I enjoyed the first lines of the book the best:

> When we were kids, Mother never let us have coloring books. She said they were bad for us because they taught us to only see that which is inside the lines. You don't need anyone telling you how or where you should color. Draw outside the lines.[10]

I hear this as another way of saying to follow the path that God has laid out for you. Keep your eyes on Jesus, the light, and don't look at the lines that the world draws for you.

Sunday, Hilary ate 840 calories and 13 oz. of fluid. Celebration time! We took a walk on the sky bridge and heard some Christmas carolers. They were just finishing, but sang one more song for us, because we had only just arrived. It was so very wonderful. I could see Pearl Dumars, EJay and Jim Weber, Harland Wendt, Rhonda Randal, and all our Richland neighbors who watched us carol them. Hilary and I hope to get our family to carol on 5C floor when it gets closer to Christmas. There are decorations everywhere, but even with all that beauty, I'm having trouble getting into the Christmas mood.

Bob and Susie came to decorate our apartment. Their decorations are better than any I could ever do. It is just beautiful. My attitude of preparing in the midst of anxiety to receive the message of peace and hope that the Jesus of Christmas represents will require more prayer time. Isn't it nice that we have Jesus, our peace and our hope, all year and not just at Christmas? Maybe I'm in Christmas all the time, and so to get more Christmas spirit just can't be possible. I'm rambling again. I'm considering deleting most of this, but since it is food for thought, you get to delete it. Have fun.

Oh, I just read a book about a study of oligoprocyanidins (OPCs, a type of bioflavonoids) in Japan. They used the OPC in barley bran to heal leukemia. Exciting news. Too bad Market America doesn't sell barley bran in a pill. Hilary would be just tickled to take another pill. I need to stop typing this rambling e-mail and start typing Tony's school paper.

Love,

Jan

Chapter 7

Hilary, Tuesday

Hilary update
Tuesday, 10 December 2002

Great news. If Hilary can drink one and a half liters of fluids, she can return to the apartment tomorrow! She is doing great. Her counts are normal. They took the PICC line out yesterday, so now she just has the central line in. All the medicines can be taken as pills (which she doesn't like to take), so she won't need a pump for IVs. The only side effect that is showing now, besides being so skinny, is very red hands and feet. The palms of her hands and the bottoms of her feet are red, burning, and itchy. This is a reaction to the last chemo that she had. We rub triamcinolone acetonide cream on them and wrap them, and they feel much better.

Thank you for your prayers.

Love,

Jan

Love, Jan

HOSPITAL DEPARTURE

Hilary update, Tuesday evening
Wednesday, 11 December 2002

Hilary is coming to the apartment tomorrow for sure! She is feeling great. The doctors told her that if she couldn't get enough fluids in, they would request an IV infusion here at home. We still have the pump. All of Hilary's medicines are now in an oral form, so we won't need the pump for anything else. No more "shake and bake" antifungal stuff. They changed that to something a little gentler on the stomach when she was fighting the nausea. So Hilary has a few pills to take each day, which she absolutely *loves* to do. Ha, ha, ha. She would rather have the IV meds.

Tonight Tony and I packed six full shopping bags out of the hospital room. We took all her clothes, except for what she plans to wear tomorrow. I suppose if they told her she would have to stay another day, her response would be, "Sorry, I can't. I don't have any clean clothes to wear, and hospital garb is out of the question!"

Tony and I plan to come to Richland tomorrow, so Irene and Hilary will have the apartment to themselves. Tony needs to work on some things on the ranch. I hope to visit school on Friday (watch the Christmas program rehearsal), and then we will return to Portland by Friday evening.
Love,
Jan

BORING

Hilary update, Sunday
Monday, 16 December 2002

"No news is good news"! Hilary is doing great. She went to clinic last Friday and has another clinic day on Tuesday. They check her blood and then give some fluids plus added minerals or other stuff that is low.

"Boring" is the word. Isn't it great? I'm not sure how often she will need to go to clinic, but probably twice a week for a while. She has moved her pill-taking to evening, so the nausea medicine will just help her sleep through the night instead of causing her to sleep all day. She is trying to eat lots, as well as follow directions to help her stay well.

Peggy came to visit. A Thanksgiving/Christmas trip. It is always like a vacation when people you love (and don't see often) are around. You don't need a noted calendar holiday to make it extra special. Elizabeth is here and Gabrielle will be here by the end of the week. We will spend Christmas at the apartment here in Portland. After Christmas, I will return to work.

Phyllis is gaining a little every day. It was very nice to visit with her and Dad this last week. Even though Phyllis can't say a word, she is still very demonstrative with her hand, body, and facial expressions. Dad was complaining about having to watch her TV shows. Phyllis made some noise and then Dad said, "Oh, I know I like ninety percent of all the shows you like." She nodded her head and grinned. We all laughed.

We've watched *Lord of the Rings* again today. I've probably seen this movie six times. Elizabeth shared a thought from J. R. R. Tolkien's *Lord of the Rings:* "Not all those who wander are lost."[11] Isn't this a great sentence for anyone whose lives are in a transition? We all have wandering times. I know the Light of Christmas is helping my wandering times.

Blessings to all of you.

Love,
Jan

SKIN BIOPSIES

Hilary update, day 26: Hope
Wednesday, 18 December 2002

Yesterday we went to clinic, and something hopeful happened. Hilary was sent to the dermatologist to have some skin biopsies taken. They

Love, Jan

were checking for GVH. If some GVH is present, then Hilary won't have to do the transplant with the cord blood from Germany. It will be very unlikely that GVH is present, but not impossible. I have been praying for this miracle of GVH.

When I told Dr. Simic that I was praying for some GVH, she told me that it was not probable. She did not want to give me false hope. But as Linda says, it is not hope in an action, but hope in Jesus, whom we trust to take care of us. We will know of the results in about a week.

Hope. What an exciting emotion. I know that Dr. Simic doesn't want us to be disappointed if our hope doesn't produce the results we want. But even though we are hoping for some GVH, our trust in Jesus will cover any disappointment that might occur. We can then hope with great excitement, because the outcome doesn't really matter. How fun!

Love,
Jan

COMING TO RICHLAND

Last Hilary update for 2002
Friday, 27 December 2002

No news is good news. Our wonderful boring lives are boring. One piece of information is the results of the skin biopsy. The rash is *not* caused by GVH. The rash must be caused by prescription drugs, soaps, or leftover chemo. Who knows?

When we found out, I said, "Darn, darn! We were hoping for some GVH so we would be done with all of this."

Susan, the nurse practitioner, said, "Maybe you are done."

This was said casually and I didn't jump on her words like a hungry fox on a rabbit, but just soaked them in like a desert rain. Hilary has an appointment with Dr. Fleming on Tuesday the 7th. She'll learn more then. Help us pray for wisdom. Wisdom for Dr. Fleming and wisdom for Hilary. Up until now, we just did what we were told to do; now Hilary has to decide if she needs to proceed with the cord blood. We need to follow the Light, not man's wisdom. And I want the easy way out, which isn't always the path that we are to follow.

Today, Hilary is dog-sitting Sean and Nicky's new pug puppy. He is so cute and so little. He is only six weeks old, weighing around three pounds. He is so small that he doesn't look like a dog. He likes to sit around my feet as I type this letter. I'm being careful where I put my feet. He hides under the computer table and then he crawls out to investigate. He has slept with Hilary off and on all day. She would really like to get a dog, but this apartment won't allow pets. Too bad. This puppy is so cute!

Our Christmas was very nice. We started on Christmas Eve with some caroling at the clinic and 5C floor. Deb, Del, and Teisha joined us, which made our singing much better. Then we ate lunch at a lovely Indian restaurant. I'm not much on curry, but the food was very good. After all the work of singing and then eating such tastes, we came home and took a long nap. Irene was the only worker and stood in line for a honey-baked ham. After she got home, she also took a nap.

When we got moving again around 6:00, Tony and I went to buy some potatoes and found all the grocery stores closed. No problem—we would just get the potatoes at a store that would be open on Christmas Day. Something would be open. If the Hitching Post stayed open for part of Christmas Day, something in Portland would be open. So after early Mass, we went looking again for a store that would carry potatoes. No luck. Irene was devastated that our Christmas dinner would be a failure. I said that we could have carrots and celery—we didn't need potatoes. Gabrielle left the kitchen to separate the gifts. Elizabeth told me not to be so cheerful. Hilary hid from the tension and didn't say anything. Tony saved the day by borrowing some potatoes from Mike and Shelly. It's a good thing we have Tony around!

Our dinner was wonderful. The gifts were abundant and we all had wonderful naps, great visiting, then watched a couple of movies. I wanted to play some games, but we didn't have enough energy. It was just a wonderful day of rest. Then on the 26th, we went to Albany to visit some of Tony's family. Sue and Gary were down from Alaska, and Lizzy was home from Australia. We had a great visit!

Tomorrow, we plan to travel to Richland. I'm praying that Hilary doesn't get sick! We have the blessings of OHSU to go to Richland, but we still need to be careful because Hilary's immune system is immature. Her counts are good, and she is promising to eat and drink properly, so home we come! We're excited and nervous all at the same time. Hilary wants to visit people, but "careful" is the big word. I'm asking that if you wish to visit, please call first and I will ask you about your health. Yet, Hilary wants to go to a ball game, to church, etc.

We are certainly going to be testing Gabe's stem cells. Hilary wants to be as normal as possible. She doesn't like being talked about and treated like a cancer victim. Be sure to bring stories about yourselves. Gabrielle will be coming with Todd either Sunday or Monday. Irene has to work, so she will be staying in Portland. It will be just Elizabeth, Tony, Hilary and me arriving Saturday night. Exciting...scary.

... I hope we have good roads.

... I feel like I did when I put the girls on the school bus for the first time.

... There is something safe about a hospital.

... Is my house safe?

... Couldn't somebody paint virus blue so we could all see them and stay away?

... Help, I'm no longer in control.

.... Who said you were ever in control anyway?

... OK, deep breath.

... Jesus, my daily bread, help me trust in your protection...

See you soon,

Love,

Jan

LIFE UPDATE

Hilary update
Monday, 06 January 2003

Many people have commented about how much they enjoy our e-mails, but I'm hoping our updates will be much further apart. It is not that we don't need your prayers anymore, or that we love you any less, it is because we hope our lives will be so boring that an e-mail would just clutter your inbox like some junk mail.

I will write tomorrow about Hilary's trip to clinic. I'm thinking that Dr. Fleming will explain suggestions for Hilary's further health plans. Right now, Hilary is doing very well. She is getting stronger every day. Our trip home was blessed. Hilary went to church and attended two basketball games. She had visitors every day either by phone (because they had a cold) or in person. Be assured, when or if some news arrives within this journey of the leukemia battle, I will certainly e-mail with vigor.

I know that your prayers have been important warriors in our fight. Steve Shold asked me once why I thought prayers were so important. I just know, or I have learned during this process, that prayers are tangible, and they are powerful. He commented that if God were all-knowing, then God already knew our needs, and so why would we need to pray? (Of course, being the wonderful teacher Steve is, he already had an answer for his questions. He was just wondering about my thinking process.) So, in agreement with Steve, I am ending this e-mail with a thought from Stephen Verney that prayer is not us trying to grab hold of God but that prayer is recognizing God coming to us. Isn't that well said?

Love to you all,
Jan

P.S. Keep praying.

Love, Jan

TUESDAY VISIT WITH DR. FLEMING

Hilary update
Wednesday, 08 January 2003

Dr. Fleming continues to recommend transplant with the cord blood from Germany. This team of doctors wants Hilary to live with confidence and no fear of a returning leukemia. With Gabe's stem cells, every time Hilary gets sick, she will wonder if it is cancer. (I think that might happen anyway.) Hilary will have another appointment on the 21st with a bone marrow test and another CAT scan. They are checking the health of the marrow and health of the lungs. If they find any leukemia or fungus, the battle will have to heat up fast. I'm confident both are long gone. The next transplant will be in a couple of months or longer. Hilary needs to gain weight and strength. Thanks for your continued prayers.

Love,
Jan

TWO WEEKS LATER

Hilary update, January 21
Wednesday, 22 January 2003

I've missed writing to everyone. In truth, I miss hearing from everyone. When I don't write, I don't get any messages. As they say, "We get what we give," "Treat other people as you want to be treated," "What goes around comes around," etc.

Hilary had a clinic appointment yesterday. She had a CAT scan to check the fungus, and a bone marrow test to check for leukemia. We should have the results in a week. Hilary doesn't have to go back to clinic for three weeks. No more blood tests, unless something shows up with today's tests. She weighs 105 pounds, so that is an increase!

98

Hip, hip, hooray! They don't want to jump into the next stem cell transplant until they are confident that there is no little fungus floating around. It must take a lot of time for the body to clear away those little bugs.

I keep hoping Dr. Fleming will change his mind about the cord blood transplant. Hilary says, "Just keep on hoping, Mom," and pats me on my shoulder. It is the same look I give kids in my classroom when they hope for an "A" without studying.

Hilary is living a normal life, which includes eating out, and going to movies and church, and she even plans to fly to California to visit Aunt Peggy soon. Last weekend we went to the beach for an afternoon. When the sunset began, everyone stopped and faced the ocean. It was like the whole world had stopped for a few minutes. No one was walking. Very neat! You know, driving to the beach from the apartment is like driving to La Grande from Richland. Why do we think it is so far?

As Elizabeth and I were coming home from Portland on Monday, I caught myself in my old habit of "worry." I was so grateful for the clear, spring-like roads and then I worried about what summer weather was going to be. Oh, what little faith I have! I can only live each day as it is given to me and trust Jesus to take care of the rest. I wonder how many times that lesson will have to be re-taught to my slow brain for it to really take hold. "This day our daily bread."

I had another reminder lesson. Last Thursday I drove over a rock with my car and ripped a hole in the oil pan (plus other stuff). I was so disgusted with myself! I coasted into the Sholds' driveway, and Steve not only brought me home, but he is taking time to tinker with my broken car. My main mechanic is in Portland taking a CNA (Certified Nursing Assistant) class. When I dropped off car parts last night, Millie gave me soup for my supper. I am reminded again that we are not an island when we are part of the body of Christ. I have felt that special *holding* for many months now. Thank you.

Love, Jan

Hope this finds each one of you living a *normal* life which includes eating out, seeing some movies, going to church, visiting family and friends, being a friend for someone who has hit a rock, and stopping to view a beautiful sight created by God.

Love to all of you.

Jan

ONE WEEK LATER

Hilary update
Tuesday, 04 February 2003

I've had a few messages asking about Hilary, so I thought it was time for an update.

Hilary is in California visiting my sister, Peggy, and Uncle Cal. She was to fly back to Portland last Saturday, but they are having such an enjoyable time together that Hilary changed her flight to next Monday. She has a doctor's appointment on Tuesday the 11th, or she probably would stay in California for a month. She is especially enjoying the warm, sunny days, plus the company of Aunt Peggy and Uncle Cal.

The last tests came back very normal, so we are waiting for a time frame from Dr. Fleming. Maybe we'll know more after the 11th.

I have been staying in Richland most of the time. I've enjoyed a few basketball games, cleaned a few messy corners, and read a little. I turned the TV on at noon one Saturday, just so I would have some noise in the house, and a movie came on. Then when it was over, another movie came on, so I watched it. It has been a long time since I was such a couch potato. I did feel a little guilty, but eased the guilt with advertisement work (working during the advertisements). Of course, last Saturday I was glued to the TV, watching everything about the space shuttle Columbia. Hearing about death, unforgiveness, or anger, always makes me sad.

I read today: "Is anything too hard for the Lord?" Genesis 18:14. Isn't that a wonderful question?

I'll talk with you again when I have more news.

Love,

Jan

ONE WEEK LATER

Hilary update

Tuesday, 11 February 2003

No news is good news. Nothing will happen with Hilary and the second transplant for at least another two months. They are waiting because of the fungal fight. They don't see any fungi present in the lungs, but they are being very cautious about any unseen fungus that might be hiding.

Ten years ago fungus killed many people. (Fungus is what killed Ryan.) Everyone knows that leukemia is a killing cancer, but not everyone knows that a fungal infection is as deadly as cancer. So my prayers are that the antifungal medicine and Gabrielle's transplanted immune system rids Hilary of any hiding fungus. Also, please pray that no other fungus decides that Hilary is a wonderful place to live.

Dr. Fleming said he would wait until September for the next transplant, just to fight the fungus for a long, long time, but that might be chancing a leukemia-memory-cell wakeup party. We *don't* want them to wake up! Thus, May seems to be the month for a second transplant. We'll see what March's bone marrow test tells us. March is 100 days past Gabe's stem cell transplant. One hundred days seems to be a mile marker. (I know that we celebrate 100 days of school!)

Interesting thought: I've noticed that it seems easier to pray when a small crisis is at hand. If I'm in a large crisis, I cannot pray at all. But, if I'm coasting along in normal living, I also find myself not focused in prayer life. I sure don't like crisis in my life, but I do like the prayer communion I have when that happens. What a conflict! Please know that I am continuing to pray for all of you (but I'm coasting in normal living, so that tells you what kind of prayers you're getting. Sorry...)

I'm working to pray in a deeper way, so I can have that prayer communion during normal living. Patty, my car partner, is reading a book to me called *Praying Self-Abandonment to Divine Love* by Slawomir Biela. It is full of great thoughts that Patty and I are both enjoying. Yet, reading a book about prayer is like reading a book about dieting and hoping you'll lose weight. Application is the hardest and most important part!

Hope this finds all of you in a "no news is good news" mode and that your prayer life is fun-filled visiting with Jesus!

Love always,
Jan

DECISION APPOINTMENT

Hilary update, March 11
Thursday, 13 March 2003

Tuesday morning: Good morning. Today is a clinic day for Hilary. We are expecting healthy news. She is gaining weight, growing hair, and is healthy enough to catch a cold (because she is running around to social events like normal healthy people do). Wonderful!

Tony and I came down so we could go with Hilary to this doctor visit. Everyone seems just fine with Hilary having another transplant, except me. I'm getting used to the idea, but I still have this "No! No! No!" feeling. I don't want Hilary to have doubts about doing another transplant, but I also need to have peace about her having another transplant. I'm hopeful that with more information, I'll leave today with confidence that we are doing the right thing. Anyway, my questions basically come to one thing: Are we trading a maybe return of leukemia for a lifetime of GVH? Which philosophy is best for Hilary's situation: "A stitch in time saves nine," or "Don't fix something that isn't broken"? As I've pondered these viewpoints for over a month, I have received different messages from different people.

Here are some of your thoughts that keep rolling around in my head:

Sandra's: "Honor the doctor with the honor that is his due in return for his services; for he too has been created by the Lord. Healing itself comes from the Most High, like a gift from a king." (Ecc. 38:1–2 JB)

Peggy's naturopath: "Since you are using a matching cord blood, go with it! It will not carry much GVH problems because it is immature stem cells and will become exactly what she needs."

Toni Nickles: "My brother had a transplant last fall and he is now getting his second transplant. It seems to be a common practice in Seattle and Los Angeles."

And, of course, I hear God say: "What makes you think that I'm going to desert Hilary now?"

With all of that, why am I still so hesitant and frightened? It is not that I don't trust God; it is that I don't trust our ability to listen to God. Do these doctors pray about their decisions? God gives us brains to make choices. These choices *always* have consequences. What is God's truth for Hilary's life? I'm confident Hilary will live; I just don't want her life to be hampered by a horrible GVH problem. How bad is this problem going to be? Only God knows. Maybe it would be better to wait?

I'm hoping Dr. Fleming can give me enough information so that I can have peace about all of this. This is silly of me to be so confused, but when they were forced to use Gabrielle's stem cells because of the fungus, I felt that God had intervened and changed their plans so Hilary would have the best solution. I hate to mess up that best solution. Am I wrong in thinking these thoughts?

This confusion needs to stop. That is why I am here today. My prayer now is that I am able to express these concerns with a calm voice and

I won't shake Hilary's trust and faith with my questions. I've gotten her permission to ask my questions and I've shared my questions with her. I didn't want her to be surprised when I ask Dr. Fleming. I have learned that my mouth gets me in trouble more than any other thing. It is words I say and words I fail to say that mess me up all the time. I don't want that to happen today!

Well, now that I've taken all your time voicing my questions and have used your e-mail space for my journaling, I'll close and finish this letter later with real facts of the doctor appointment.

P.S. Toni Nickle's brother is receiving his stem cell transplant today. Say a prayer for him, please.

Wednesday morning:

Well, Dr. Fleming checked Hilary over and was concerned about the cough/cold. Hilary assured him that it was a different cough than the fungus cough. After the exam, I asked my first question, "Are you still planning to do a second transplant in May?"

Then, Dr. Fleming expressed the same questions and concerns that I was having. I was so surprised. I didn't need to ask any of the other questions I had written down.

Apparently, Dr. Maziars, who is head of the department, is asking, "What if we already have a cure?" They don't want to jump into anything with the fungus still a possible problem. They are just as worried about the fungus as the leukemia! The earliest they will do anything is June, unless the leukemia shows up. Then, in June they might decide to wait until September.

The longer they wait, the better they feel about the fungus problem. Dr. Fleming did say that Hilary was in a class of her own. They don't have enough data about people using an identical twin stem cell transplant, surviving a fungal infection, and starting with sixteen chromosomes affected by leukemia. Certainly, without Gabrielle, Hilary would not be alive right now. Apparently, people just don't survive what Hilary has already survived. (That sounds like something God is involved with, doesn't it?) Anyway, they don't know what to do.

Dr. Fleming indicated that we could go anywhere for a second opinion. In fact, I think he would really like to hear another voice about the next step for Hilary. They are certainly split at OHSU for Hilary's next-step plan. Dr. Fleming was surprised that Dr. Maziars is being so conservative. Usually, he said, he (Dr. Fleming) was the conservative one.

I do know one thing: they are worried about leukemia and fungus, not GVH. They'll cross the bridge of GVH after the fungus/leukemia is no longer a concern. I also learned they've decided the cord blood would not be a good choice because cord blood usually takes thirty days to engraft. They are worried that the fungus might show up on day 15, then, with no engraftment, a very ugly picture would occur. Thus, they have started another search within the world donor bank for an adult donor. Please tell everyone you know to join the bone marrow donor program! So many decisions!

Hilary had a bone marrow biopsy. I'm anxious to hear the results of that test.

We appreciate all your continued prayers! How can we thank you enough? They are the support that gets us to the table so we can continue feeding on "our daily bread"! Thank you.

Love to all of you,

Jan

SPRING

Hilary update, March 20
Thursday, 20 March 2003

Today is the first day of spring. (I always thought spring started on March 21, but the local news broadcast informed me that today is the shifting of a new season.) Yesterday, Hilary got her central line removed.

Love, Jan

I asked her if she now felt normal. She informed me that she has always felt normal.

The first look at the bone marrow biopsy said that Hilary's bone marrow is clear of leukemia. Praise God! I was so worried that the leukemia had returned. Hilary's white count was low and that was one of the reasons for the first bone marrow biopsy in Alaska. It was difficult to return to work on Wednesday morning after leaving Hilary at her appointment on Tuesday. Fortunately, I have some wonderful teaching partners and they prayed with and for me, and my week continued with a clear mind, knowing that God has everything in control.

I also thank you for praying for us. Your prayers are truly important! Now we all need to pray for our troops and wisdom for our leaders. Should we ever think that we are not important because we are not in a position of leadership? I think not. We have the most important job of all: prayer! Thanks for your faithful prayers for us.

Love,

Jan

Easter Greetings

Hilary update
Sunday, 27 April 2003

Here we are, one week from Easter and, after receiving many inquiries about Hilary, I determined it's time to do another update. Hilary is doing great! We still don't know our next step. Even though we've been trying to set a date for a second opinion appointment in Seattle, nothing is planned yet. So, as you have guessed, no news is good news.

I have one story from last weekend. Hilary jumped into the car after hurrying from a restaurant and said, "I felt the wind blowing my hair." She then pulled down the visor to look in the mirror and exclaimed, "And it is standing straight up." I looked at her and chuckled. Her hair is only a quarter of an inch long and if anyone looked at her, I'm sure they would only notice the length, not that it was standing up.

Hilary and Irene are moving to a newer, brighter, bigger apartment than the one Peggy and I found in a three-day quick search. I think they will be completely moved in before the first of May. Elizabeth is helping them paint, Tony is helping them lift, Pat is loaning them a pickup, Sean and Nicky are helping them with boxes, etc. Irene wants to return all the borrowed furniture. I see the new apartment as another statement of "Hilary is well and we need to move on."

Our Easter was wonderful. We stood through church because there was standing room only. The music was awesome, the sermon was OK, the people were beautiful (we were standing by the side wall so we could see people's faces and had to turn sideways to see the altar). I thought of how different this Easter was compared to sunrise service on the hill and breakfast at the school, but I truly enjoyed being with my girls even if I missed my church family at home. When we were a couple of blocks away from our services, I saw people with black leather jackets, baggy pants, and purple hair. I wondered if they were our society's self-made lepers. I realize that clothes do not imply the heart of a person, but the people at church were dressed strikingly different than the black, baggy and purple. I plan to read about the ten lepers. I want to know: did those ten lepers just "happen" upon Jesus, or did they search him out? Why do some of us search for Jesus while others don't? How do we explain the wonderment of Jesus? I've decided it's over my head. It is a mystery.

I hope you had a wonderful Easter. Thank you for encouraging me to write. I have found that I enjoy this journaling. I hated writing in school, and now I enjoy writing to you. Another mystery. Thank you again for your prayers. I hope they bring you closer to the wonderment of Jesus.

Love to you all,

Jan

Chapter 8

NEWS

Hilary update
Sunday, 11 May 2003

We've gotten two messages this past month.

Number one: Hilary has her second opinion appointment on May 29, in Seattle. I hope, as you all know, that this doctor will encourage Hilary to wait until the leukemia shows its ugly head again before jumping into another treatment plan. As Dr. Maziars said, "We might already have a cure." We all know that if Hilary gets another transplant, she may fight GVH for the rest of her life. No one knows how bad that problem might be. Anyway, another big decision-planning day is May 29.

Number two: I am going to have a hysterectomy on May 20. I was going to keep this quiet because I didn't want to be talked about, felt sorry for, etc., but since this needs to be done before school is out, everyone will know. I'll miss the last couple of weeks with my class, which really bothers me. I am planning to be there the last day, if I have to crawl into that classroom.

Love, Jan

Thanks to your prayers, this class has improved beyond my expectations. I am truly sending on a totally different class than the one I received. I just wish I had a few more weeks with them. Oh, well, I have to remember that for everything there is a season, God is in control of all seasons, and my season with these students is finished. I remember that I invited Jesus to help me teach this class in the beginning. Do you remember me asking you to pray for this class? Then I am amazed at the outcome? Oh what little faith I have! Hope you had some wonderful Mother's Day celebrations. Thank you again for all your prayers!

Love,

Jan

SEATTLE APPOINTMENT

Hilary update
Friday, 30 May 2003

What an interesting, stressful day! We left Portland around 6:00 A.M. to arrive in time for Hilary's appointment. It was clear, with the promise of a hot day ahead. The farther north we traveled, the colder it became. We started with the vent blowing in the car and ended with the heater moving the air around. The traffic was absolutely horrible. I can't believe people drive in that crowd every day!

We met with a team of doctors from Seattle. The lead doctor did an excellent job, using a white board to share statistics, and he even drew some pictures to explain everything. Hilary's plan is: search the international bank again to find a donor, continue to check very carefully for any leukemia signs, and then decide about a second transplant when we find a perfect matching donor. What stressed me was the misconception that we planned to move our treatment to them. I did feel like I was in the presence of a car salesman—a small round table, white board with numbers on it, windowless room, etc. I think Hilary's stress came from all the statistics plus the idea that she should move away from the care of OHSU.

Peggy took excellent notes and Irene asked some excellent questions. Tony stayed home because of a scheduling problem, and when we tried to explain everything to him using Hilary's cell phone in our car ride home, we all disagreed about some of the information Peggy wrote down. That's why whenever people do things like this, the more ears that are available, the better the information is received. I do wish Tony had been there to hear it firsthand. No one thought this meeting would upset all of us.

Here is some of the data we learned: Seattle has a 20 percent higher success rate than OHSU. That's big! There is a 10 percent chance that Hilary is already cured. Pretty low. If we needed to transplant again, and we used Gabe again, Hilary would only have a 50 percent chance of not relapsing. If she used an unrelated donor, she would have a 5 percent chance of relapsing. Problem is, when you use an unrelated donor, you have a 70 percent chance of graft versus host disease (GVHD),[11] which has risk. Dr. Raddich stressed that we really should decide where to do the second transplant, because the facility doing the stem cell search should also do the transplant.

Hilary got all blotchy on the face and looked as if she was going to cry (which she probably did when she went to the bathroom). Her main comment was, "I'm going to have to wait for another three to five years before I can ever go to school."

Peggy and I both told her to go ahead and start. All of humanity moves through life as if they have years to accomplish goals, but life stops many of us from those lifelong goals via accidents, illnesses, and emergencies that are never planned for. Hilary is just beginning her school goal with the knowledge that we only live one day at a time and an evil leukemia cell can change any best-laid plans.

When we got back to the apartment, I looked up transplant information on the Internet. It might surprise some of you that this was the first time I'd checked out information using the Internet. When Hilary was first diagnosed, I tried to look for information about leukemia, and it was so overwhelming that I stopped. I needed my energy to trust and pray, not to doubt and question every move of the doctors. Anyway, Seattle does have a 20 percent higher success rate with transplant patients. I want to know why! Plus, if all these hospitals use the same bone marrow bank, why should it matter who requests a search?

Hilary has a call in to Dr. Fleming, but hasn't heard back yet. We're going to e-mail Dr. Raddich with these questions again and see what he says. When we asked in Seattle for the cause of the higher success rate, he praised the nurses. Experience is huge. But comfort and trust are also huge. We all came away with more questions than answers. Isn't that always the way things happen?

Anyway, my prayer now is: if Hilary is cured using Gabe's stem cells, no donor will be found to confuse us. But, if Hilary is to have a second transplant, a perfect donor will be available when the time comes. It is so easy for me to worry! I need to remember where I should spend my time and energy during my daily tasks. When the wind blows my boat around, I need to let go of the side and reach toward the hand that calms the wind and provides peace. It is amazing that he is always there when I truly take time to pray. That's why I need those six hours of driving between Richland and Portland. Sometimes it takes me that much time of yelling before I have the courage to let go and listen. Only then does peace enter my body, and what a blessed calm it is! It is an amazing love that truly passes all understanding. Plus the "communion of saints" is a part of all this mystery, which is a part of your prayers. Anyway, my discussion with my friend Jesus never stops.

Other news: I'm getting stronger every day.

Love to all of you! Hope the wind is calm in your life.

Love,

Jan

E-MAIL TO PEGGY

May 31, 2003

Hi, Peggy,

Thanks again for coming up and staying with me. We called Elizabeth five minutes after you called us and Elizabeth was in tears again. "I thought we were finished with this disease."

It does concern me that Hilary is so tired! She felt warm to me last night so I had her take her temperature and it was only 99.1, but that is a little high. If she starts throwing up, I'm going to be really scared! I've been praying all night about healing and I'm nervous. With Hilary's energy level, I'm not sure she can go to school.

Dr. Fleming called around 4:00 yesterday afternoon. I'm glad we were here to receive the call. I'm not sure that if we were on the road, the call would have come in. Anyway, Hilary is going to have a conference call on Tuesday. Fleming was surprised and disappointed that the doctor in Seattle told us that Seattle had a 20 percent higher success rate. Dr. Fleming said, "We are not far behind." He also said, "Hilary, you will respond the same to the treatment whether you are in Seattle or Portland. Your success rate will be the same wherever you go."

Of course, during their twenty-minute conversation we were in the middle of a plant nursery, so I only heard pieces of Hilary's part of the conversation, and of course none of Dr. Fleming's comments.

I'm not feeling at peace right now. I'm wishing I felt better/normal. I wish I had some answers/wisdom for Hilary. I need a vacation from my mind and body. I'll maybe get that when I'm able to walk down my road at home. Maybe I need to go to the beach.

Thanks for listening to my worries!

Jan

Love, Jan

HOTMAIL

Hilary update
Monday, 09 June 2003

I'm having an awful time with my Hotmail address. I can only send thirty messages in a twenty-four-hour period, and I have close to seventy-five people on my address list. Thus, it takes me three days to send one Hilary update.

Hilary is setting up an appointment with Dr. Maziars, who is the head of the department at OHSU, about doing a second transplant. He has been very hesitant about jumping into another transplant situation and asked Dr. Fleming to "prove that Hilary isn't already cured after using Gabrielle's stem cells." Of course Dr. Fleming's proof was for us to get a second opinion at Seattle, which agreed with Fleming's choice of "next step." If Maziars still is hesitant, Hilary is planning to move to Seattle to search for a new donor. My prayer is still for God to only allow a donor to materialize if Hilary needs a second transplant. Plus, the donor needs to be absolutely perfect, but not as perfect as Gabrielle!

Within one day of bending your ear while sharing my worries and fears using e-mail, I have again peace and courage. It is a testimony of the power of prayer, of your prayers. Thank you for loving us enough to pray for us, and I thank Jesus for loving us enough to give us peace and courage.

Well, here I go trying to send this to you. Some of you will get this today, some of you will get this tomorrow, some of you will get this on Wednesday, some of you will get this twice because I forgot where I stopped in my address list, some of you may never receive this email, and some of you may delete this email without even opening it because you are too kind to ask me to delete your name from my list. Oh, well. Isn't e-mail wonderful? Just think of those Oregon Trail travelers in the 1850s: they got a letter from family maybe once a year (which they kept

in special places to read again and again), no forwards or junk mail. They treasured each letter. I'm glad I have e-mail!
Love you,
Jan

DR. MAZIARS APPOINTMENT

Hilary update
20 June 2003

On Wednesday, Hilary, Irene, Gabrielle, and Todd went to visit with Dr. Maziars. They took a tape recorder with them so we could listen again to any part of the meeting that was confusing (a great suggestion from Mark and Terry). The report given to us Eastern Oregon inhabitants, with a three-way call to Aunt Peggy in California, went much better than the one in Seattle.

Irene said this meeting was much more comfortable—a large window, no white board, no table, just all of them sitting in chairs discussing different options. Maziars feels that Hilary is already past that 10 percent mark of cure because she has stayed in remission for six months. Twenty-five percent of twin-transplant patients never get into remission, so Hilary is moving up that ladder of survival. However, he is certainly open to looking for another donor, to fight the demon leukemia should it recur.

OHSU is also looking for a lab to do further testing on "high-resolution" typing. Right now, OHSU looks at 1 cell out of 500 for any leukemia signs, but they are searching for a lab that will look at 1 in 10,000 cells. This will help determine an earlier notice of any relapse. Because our health insurance doesn't pay for the donor search, OHSU needs our permission to do another look instead of jumping ahead. We said yes, please look, search, explore, and hunt for a perfect matching donor. We've had wonderful people donate money for just this purpose of "beyond insurance costs." If Hilary relapses before a donor is found, Maziars is not against using the cord blood from Germany. He doesn't think we need to worry about the fungus at this time.

Of course, Todd said, "I don't think Hilary will need another transplant." Gabrielle said, "My cells are just fine."

God is in control. If a second transplant is needed, a donor will be found, or the cord blood will be perfect for Hilary. If a second transplant is NOT needed, no matching donor will be discovered. Tomorrow is truly in God's hands, and when we let Jesus in our boat to calm the storm, why should we worry? I can say this so easily right now when the winds are not blowing. Right now the winds are still, the sky is sunny, and the fish are plentiful. Life is good!

Please pray for a friend in Eagle Creek who was just told she has an inoperable cancerous tumor close to her lung and heart. She has asked for prayers, and you are the prayer network I have. Help me pray for her!

There seems to be many people who are in need of God's peace or knowledge of his love. Know that I pray for God's blessings in your lives. Your prayers have certainly blessed us!

Love you,

Jan

LETTER FROM SEATTLE TO OHSU

Sunday, 22 June 2003

Hilary received a copy of the letter the Seattle doctor sent to Fleming about our appointment in Seattle. There were a couple of points I thought you would be interested in:

1. The unrelated-donor registry shows eleven broad matches with Hilary. One of them may end up being a complete match. However, the patient needs more high-resolution typing in order

to completely assess the suitability of the donor. Dr. Maziars is still looking for a lab that will do that high-resolution typing.

2. The experience with allogeneic transplants (stem cells from other people) following autologous transplants (stem cells from self) should be similar to syngeneic (stem cells from a twin). "Allogeneic have been written up by our center in *Biology Bone & Marrow Transplantations* 6:272, 2000. Of the 24 AML patients transplanted, 10 are alive, breaking this up by age in the 10–20 range, two of four patients were disease-free survivors." Of course, Tony says to quit comparing syngeneic (identical twin) transplants with allogeneic because there has to be a difference. We were told the chances of Gabe getting leukemia is only 5 percent higher than the general population. Thus, shouldn't a twin transplant be better than an allogeneic?

3. Ending side note: "This is obviously a very difficult case and we would be happy to help in any way in making this decision easier. I hope we have the luxury of readdressing the debates between the different types of transplants in the situation of her being in remission with a donor."

Because of Elizabeth's schedule, we have only three days here in Portland. Our list is much too long for our three days, so we are now in the process of prioritizing. I think Hilary and Gabe are going to Riddle, instead of Eliz and me, to get the car over the 4th of July.

Did you know that Grandma Bonn is giving us her old car? Tony and I have been shopping for a car, because we weren't sure about the safety of Tony driving the pickup to Ontario this winter. Then we decided we needed to use our money for house repairs instead of a car purchase. Last week, Grandma decided to buy a new car and gave us her old one. Isn't that wonderful! Time and time again, when I have wanted a "thing" and have mentioned it to God—after which I decide that I couldn't afford it and it would just wait until a different time to purchase the "thing"—Grandma would just send it over. It was always used, but I am truly amazed that my "thing" has arrived as a gift even when I knew I didn't really need it. Then I feel a bit guilty that I've visited with the Creator of the Universe about such a minor item, a "thing," and I get it. I want to clarify that I don't always get the things I visit with God about, but I get enough of those things that I know God is certainly real and listens to me.

Bill Shield has mentioned, "Coincidences happen when I pray, and when I don't pray coincidences don't happen." It reminds me of Psalm 37:4 (NIV), where David says, about God, "He will give you the desires of our hearts." If God gives us a car through Grandma, won't he allow Gabe's stem cells to be the cure for Hilary? That prayer is much more important than having a car. And I think the car is just another reminder of how much he loves us and wants to provide for us, His children. Isn't all of this awesome to think about?

Side note: we're going to let the girls have Grandma's car in Portland and Tony is still planning to drive the pickup this winter. I'll write again soon.

Love,
Jan

Chapter 9

HEADACHES

Hilary update, July 25
Friday, 25 July 2003

Surprises never cease! Even the OHSU oncology staff is stunned and shocked!

Hilary has been having horrible headaches the last two weeks. Then for the last five days, she has vomited each morning (sometimes twice a day; today she hit three). Gabrielle and Todd took her to the clinic on Tuesday. I was sure she needed air conditioning in their apartment. Something was causing the headaches! Then Thursday, yesterday, Irene took Hilary to the clinic and they admitted her to the hospital. They wanted to do some tests to explore the headache causes. First test was a CAT scan. They found a mass. So they did an MRI. The mass is 3–4 cm in diameter, in her right ventricle crossing over to the central ventricle. They plan to do brain surgery within the next three days, whenever the operating room (OR) has space, time, etc. They may even do surgery tonight, but I think Monday is probably the more likely time. They don't have a clue as to what it is. It could be leukemia-caused, but Hilary doesn't have any leukemia in the bone marrow or blood.

Irene just came in and said the neurosurgeon came to see Hilary (I missed meeting her, darn, darn, darn!). She said they will not do surgery because the tumor is deep in the brain tissue, and removing it could cause Hilary to lose strength on her left side permanently. They will only remove it if they have to. They are going to do a biopsy on Monday to determine what they/we are fighting—lymphoma from the leukemia, infection, fungus, or tumor from something unrelated. Hilary will be moved to ICU this weekend to monitor her functions and then she will be moved to Dornbecker, the children's hospital next door, because this doctor works over there. Hilary's size and age fit that OR situation.

Irene liked this doctor. I can't believe I missed her! This scares me. I feel dumb and teary-eyed.

Thank you for your continued prayers. God has not left us; he is still in control. I just don't understand why this is happening.

Jan

HEADACHE UPDATE

Hilary update
Sunday, 27 July 2003

Good morning, everyone. Hilary's headache is gone. She has been pain-free since Friday night after Judith's craniosacral therapy. Of course the medical staff thinks the reason for no headaches is steroids. However, they have stopped giving her steroids because they can mess up the biopsy test. I can think of another reason for no headaches: prayer. The doctors don't know anything about craniosacral therapy (isn't it funny that alternative medicine is unknown to the traditional doctors?), and prayer is certainly an unknown force.

When Dr. Simic and I were alone, she asked in wonderment about our seemingly calm presence in such a stressful time. I was able to say, "It is Jesus." I also told her what Hilary said last October when remission left, "Mom, don't worry! Worry only takes away the happiness that we have today." I could express that Hilary doesn't seem afraid of death or the future, and she believes we need to live each day with love, joy, and peace, not worry! (Doesn't that sound like the fruit of the Spirit?)

Yesterday was pain-free, so Elizabeth, Marissa, Irene, Hilary, and I played Phase 10 (a card game loaned to us from Debbie) for probably three hours and laughed and laughed. As far as we know, the medical staff on the oncology unit is just as surprised and stunned about this tumor as we are. It could be a lymphoma, which can be treated with steroids, chemo, and radiation. However lymphomas usually occur in people who have been on a lot of immune-suppressant drugs, which Hilary hasn't had because she had Gabe's stem cells for a transplant. It could be a fungal infection (same bad guy from the lungs), which the doctors would drain. They don't think it is a fungus, because Hilary would be a lot sicker if it were. It could be a primary brain tumor, which would be totally unrelated to leukemia. I'm not sure about the treatment of a primary brain tumor, but I think it is surgery, chemo, and radiation. They are not excited about doing surgery on Hilary because of the location of the tumor.

It could be a chloroma, which is leukemia in the brain. Leukemia normally doesn't get involved in the brain tissue—the blood brain barrier stops most leukemia. And then it could be a benign tumor, which I think is also treated with surgery. Thus, on Monday, Hilary will have a biopsy to find out what war we are fighting now. Of course, the results of the biopsy will take four to five days to arrive. Waiting is difficult, but ignorance is a nice sort of denial. They moved Hilary to ICU for monitoring. (That's where we played Phase 10, and the nurses there said it was nice to care for a patient who was laughing and playing cards.) They are very concerned about the backed-up fluid caused by the tumor, which makes pressure in the brain, which seems to have left because Hilary has no headaches now. They put on a "crown," which looked like a lifesaving ring, on her head, which will help the computer guide the brain probe during surgery. Hilary had another MRI last night to start the data of the lifesaving ring locations and tumor location. I'm really anxious to hear about the difference between last night's MRI and the one they took on Thursday night, because Hilary now doesn't have a headache. Did it move because of craniosacral therapy? Did it shrink because of steroids? Did it disappear because of prayers? Of course, this little biopsy isn't risk-free.

So, again I thank you for your continued prayers!

Friday night I had a vivid dream. I was standing in a road like Carnahan Lane, where there are two roads coming up a hill merging into one road on top. I was standing up the lane and looking down onto the two upcoming roads. There was a triangle of grass and weeds separating the two roads coming up the hill. A lady had her car parked sideways at the top of the right road as I looked down at her. The car was white and no other cars could get past it. The lady got out of her car to look around, and someone behind me yelled, "Hey lady, you're in the way." She looked toward me and said "Oh," got in her car, and moved forward just enough so both lanes were free. She was now parked at the top of the triangle of grass.

Because I don't remember many dreams, I pondered this one. I wonder if that tumor moved to the top of the triangle of grass.

On Friday, when Hilary still had a horrible headache, I opened the shower door slightly after I felt too much time had lapsed and spied her drying the floor. I told her to just leave that, don't bend over, someone else will get that, or let me do it. She said, "I didn't want anyone to slip on the wet floor." (She had at the time an elderly lady rooming with her.) It made me realize again what wonderful girls I have. Even in pain, she is thinking of other people. How can I be so blessed?

Because all of us have trials and headaches of some sort, we pray your days ahead are headache-free, or at least that the car moves far enough forward that the flow of God's blessings can reach you. You are a blessing to us. Thanks again for all your love and supportive prayers!

Love,

Jan

SURGERY

Hilary update

28 July 2003

It is now 1:45 P.M. I'm in 5C so I can write a quick update and David, one of our nurses, greeted me at the sink with, "Well, how did things go? I went upstairs earlier, and you were already in OR." This family of medical personnel is all so concerned!

Yesterday, Hilary's headache came back. It was a whopper, but she told me it was not any worse than Thursday's headache. No wonder Irene took her to the clinic and they said to admit. This headache was horrible! The ICU staff was working hard to control the pain and nausea. Morphine was the drug of choice. I dreaded waiting until this afternoon for the surgery, knowing that Hilary would be in constant pain while waiting. Then at 8:00, they told us we were moved to the first spot of the day instead of the second. I was glad but also concerned about the first person. As it turned out, person number one just didn't get to the MRI place in time to get their lifesaving-ring-crown picture, so Hilary got to go first. I think that was a God-thing.

She is now back at ICU and sleeping. The preliminary report of the biopsy is "we really don't know." It looks like a tumor that had some goopy stuff that looked like it might be fungal. I asked what kind of tumor, and they don't know. So we still are waiting to hear which of the five choices we are facing. Irene asked if it could be both, and the doctor said yes. We might be fighting two wars. That would be familiar, but not good!

Love, Jan

I woke up thinking about *hope* and reminded Hilary of Jeremiah 29:11–12, where God tells his people in Babylon that he had a future and a hope for them. They were not where they wanted to be and God gave them a promise. Hilary smiled and nodded her head. What a wonderful thing...hope...I think it is just as powerful as love. Hope is the beginning of confidence when everything looks bad.

I have visited with Jeff, whose wife first came in when Hilary was having her transplant and she is now back with lots of problems. His hope is fading. It is really sad when we lose our hope! Please join me in prayers for him and Terry, as their situation looks grim. When I was so numb on Friday night, I went for a walk on the sky bridge and saw a man that looked hopeless. As he leaned on the railing, I stopped and asked if he wanted someone to walk with him. (I thought maybe I could give him some comfort.) He told me his story, and so I told him mine, and when I had finished he told me he would pray for us. He gave me comfort instead of me helping him. I felt so bad that I had not said "I'll pray for you" first. Then I saw a new patient on 5C and she immediately said she would pray for us, and again I had not stated that sentence. I've pondered why I'm so hesitant to express "I'll pray for you," but their statements sure seemed God-given when I felt so numb!

Thank you for your prayers!

Love,

Jan

HILARY HEADACHE, WEDNESDAY

Hilary update
Thursday, 31 July 2003

Hilary is feeling great! No headache, no nausea, very little pain medication, on steroids, and no news. The pathologists still don't know

124

what the tumor is. Today's report stated that there are some dead cells in the tumor (isn't that interesting?) and the soupy stuff doesn't look fungal. (Great news. We hope it is true.) We really don't have any final report yet. Dr. Simic is calling pathology daily, I think the brain surgeon is calling them daily, and every medical person we've worked with on 5C and ICU is asking us if we have any news. They are all concerned (probably because Hilary has stolen their hearts), plus I think they want to get started on the next battle.

I appreciate all the push to find out who the enemy is, but I really thank God for how well Hilary seems today. It's days like today that make you feel this is all a big mistake. I'm glad Dr. Durram allowed us to view the MRIs of Hilary's head. We got to see the comparison from Thursday's MRI and Saturday's MRI. They looked the same, and seeing the MRIs made this tumor real. I'm sure Hilary would tell me that the headaches were very real. It's an interesting idea that this tumor may have been around for a long time with no ill effects until now. I'm glad it is not bothering Hilary today!

They moved us from ICU this morning around 3:00. We are on 5A in a small private room. We're so glad we have a private room. Monday night was a bit rough (one seizure). The ICU nurse was continually on the lookout for another stiffening spell, the sign of a seizure. They did an extra CAT scan to make sure she wasn't hemorrhaging someplace. Then, Tuesday was much better, and today Hilary seems normal.

Hilary and I reread Jeremiah 29, the letter to the exiles. They were to plant gardens, marry, have children, etc., and then in seventy years they could go home. It was interesting to read. If you haven't ever read that chapter, take a look. After we read it, Hilary decided I needed to bring in her anatomy book.

Monday, when Elizabeth and Marissa needed to go back to La Grande, Lizzy Coburn drove them to La Grande and then drove back to Portland. Elizabeth studied and Marissa slept. Lizzy is a very special cousin, roommate, and friend! How do you say thank you to such a

Love, Jan

gift of time? Aunt Margaret made some meals so Hilary wouldn't have to eat yucky hospital food. We all are enjoying those treats—another wonderful gift of time. You are all so special. Your prayers are gifts of time. Thank you.

Love,
Jan

TUMOR IS LEUKEMIA

Hilary update, August 1
03 August 2003

Good morning. Do you ever wake up with a song running through your head? My mind does that often. Usually it is a song I'm working on, but if I'm not trying to memorize a piece the song is from some old memory bank. Sometimes the song is a full orchestra playing Beethoven. Sometimes the song is a hymn. Sometimes it is a children's song. Sometimes it is only one phrase or only one line, and on those mornings I go crazy. This morning's song is a spiritual called "Wayfaring Stranger." I smiled when I recognized the song of the day. So appropriate.

We were told the results of the tumor yesterday. The enemy is leukemia. Those awful spies are hiding deep in the brain. They are enclosed and haven't infiltrated the bone marrow as far as we know, but they look exactly like they did a year ago. I didn't want this choice. I didn't want any of the choices, but I especially didn't want this one because I have a glimmer of the treatment leading to fighting this new exhibit of leukemia.

First, Hilary will need radiation to the overall brain, and extra radiation to the tumor location. Then she'll need another bone marrow transplant. They are not eager to use the cord blood from Germany because of the long engraftment period. They have only one other match from the adult list, which they have only matched broadly (the first four

126

surface proteins on the cells match). I have very little hope that a HLA match will play out completely to a perfectly matching donor, but we need to try. Hilary is so hard to match, as is true with so many other people who need a donor. This is one reason why many people use their own cleaned-up cells for a transplant.

I appreciate again the bone marrow drives we had in Baker County for Hilary. Would you please ask all your Christmas card friends if they are on the list? I wish it didn't cost anything for the average Joe to just go into the Red Cross and get their finger poked. But if there isn't a drive going on, the cost runs about $100.

When Dr. Simic was talking to us about the tumor and treatment, and answering our questions, Hilary said, "Things like this happen," which I noticed brought a slight tearing to Dr. Simic's eyes. I don't think they run into many people like Hilary. How can she be so strong? I know Irene is angry. I was disappointed. Tony is frustrated. I asked Hilary on our walk to the chapel if she was angry or sad. She said she was just annoyed.

Because I'm playing for Danielle's wedding in a week, I decided I should try to practice on the piano in the VA hospital chapel. Hilary went with me. As we were working, a gentleman came in and told us we would need to stop if someone came in needing to meditate and pray. Of course we agreed, but I thought, "And who says we are not meditating and praying while playing this piano?" I have done that task many times. Tony prays with his eyes open and I pray while I play the piano. Why is a chapel supposed to be quiet? *I like making noise!* And I don't think my loving Jesus minds at all. I think a bit of anger is following my feelings of disappointment. Who am I angry with? I don't know. Life, I guess. I ask the "why" questions and hear Hilary's "why not" responses.

I need some direction right now. I need some important task. I need guidance. Maybe I should fast.

Thanks for allowing me to vent via the Internet into your e-mail boxes. I do appreciate this opportunity to write, and while writing I get a little more focused. Thank you also for all your prayers. Could you

Love, Jan

read a little before you pray and share with me a few verses that impress you? My disappointment is making me a bit depressed.

Love to you all!

Jan

LIVER COUNTS

Hilary update
Saturday, 02 August 2003

I know this sounds strange, but we were fully expecting Hilary to be released from the hospital yesterday. I realize that it's only been a couple days since surgery, but all the radiation treatment can be completed as an outpatient procedure and Hilary is feeling well. She doesn't have any headaches. Even though she has a little stomach ache caused by the steroids, she is feeling fine. Then, we were told her liver counts were elevated. Bummer...no release.

She had an ultrasound last night. She was poked nine times in trying to get blood samples. Nothing about this hospital is fun anymore. The counts this morning were higher yet, so she is going to get another PICC line and the liver specialist is going to see her. Hilary has lost some of that wonderful attitude. Yesterday and today, Jamie, Corie, Cathy, and Holly came to visit. I know that is helping with attitude. She got moved to another room today. This is the fifth room she has been in for this hospital stay. The only thing she seems to enjoy is visitors, the book *Sea Biscuit*, and showers, which don't seem enough to cover disappointment. Disappointment can be really bad!

We need to find something to laugh about, and I'm brain dead. Talk to you later.

Love,

Jan

HILARY'S FREE SUNDAY

Hilary update
03 August 2003

Yesterday evening, Hilary's liver counts started coming down. This morning's report was lower yet. The counts are still high but we were able to escape. "Run, run, as fast as you can...."

Hilary will need to go to the clinic daily for blood tests this week, plus visit the radiologist. Then the girls want to do something, maybe a movie, but first I wanted to send a message out, because yesterday's e-mail was kind of depressing. We are moving forward. "Planting gardens" (Jer. 29:5).

Love to all of you. You are so special!

Jan

AUGUST 4 UPDATE, AND AUGUST 9 BONE MARROW DRIVE

Hilary update, August 4
05 August 2003

The apartment makes life better! Hilary needed to be at the radiologist at 8:00 A.M. for the fitting of a mask. This mask will help them point the radiation to the proper spot in her brain. There are always risks and possible side effects, but I think over all, radiation will not be as bad as chemo. Hilary looked like she wore a waffle iron when she was done. Cute.

The radiation treatments will begin on Tuesday. Her liver counts are continually moving downward. They are still really high, but at least they are moving in the right direction.

I was able to visit with Norene, the coordinator of the bone marrow search. She was wonderful. The cord blood from Germany is still available. They are doing further testing on a donor from England that matches at the broad level. When I asked about doing a bone marrow drive, she said that would be a good thing to do, because Hilary is a tough girl to match. Never knew that Tony's German history and my English history would be a tough match. Tony said, "Well, the Germans and English were always at war. No time to create any matches."

Anyway, when we got home, Irene told us that Debbie called and there is a donor drive planned for this Saturday here in Portland. Please pass on this information to anyone you know in the Portland area. There is funding for the first sixty donors, then it only costs $25 for anyone past that number. They are hoping for 100 people. I would like to see 200. Teisha might need a donor in the future and Hilary certainly hasn't found a perfect matching donor (except Gabrielle, her identical twin sister). Who knows how many other people are looking for a matching donor and cannot find one? Maybe people could carpool from the Albany or Longview areas. Make a fun day of it—go shopping, eat at a great restaurant (like the Reserve), or just laugh with your friends because you are doing something wonderful together. The rules of the game are: you need to be between the ages of eighteen and sixty and have no major health problems. I think there are other rules, but I can't think of them right now. Call the Red Cross for all those rules.

Love,

Jan

APRON STRINGS

Hilary update
Wednesday, 06 August 2003

Today was Hilary's first experience with radiation. She said it tasted like a microwave. Interesting! She has ten treatments, and then in about mid-September she will begin treatment for her second transplant. Of course, we are praying for the perfect donor for this procedure. Please encourage everyone you know to join the donor list!

Dr. Maziars is leaning toward using the cord blood from Germany, but it is mismatched on the DR marker, which is not a good place to be missing. Because it is a cord blood, they are not too worried about the mismatch. I'm not sure what to hope for. Is the cord blood a perfect donor for Hilary? Is there someone else out there who would be a better match? I think someone with no mismatched spots would be better. A perfect match would be best.

Hilary is preparing for the battle in September by eating well, sleeping a lot, exercising some. Her three-week headache caused her to lose ten pounds. She is trying to build her body for the next attack.

Because Hilary is nineteen years old and she would like the apron strings loosened, Tony and I are heading back to Richland today. Tony will stay in Richland while continuing his plans for Treasure Valley Community College and nursing school. I will come back to Portland tomorrow for Danielle's wedding and then will go to California to work on my Motives business. (I started Motives as a summer job to help me with my "empty nest.") We are *not* thrilled about leaving, but Hilary is tired of being smothered. I catch myself talking for her. Not good. I look at other girls her age who already have a year of college behind them, are working at temporary jobs, planning for career jobs, meeting new people, even meeting the possible someone they could marry, moving in their faith journey closer to God. And even though Hilary is in a unique situation, she has made it plainly understood that she wants these apron strings untied. We are still important and needed, but our position needs to move to a new level. *Wow.* Bummer! Darn! This is hard! When should we camp on her doorstep and when should we move across the state?

Grandma Bonn said we raised our children to fly from the nest, but how do you watch someone fly away when the wind is blowing so hard? Don't you hold them inside until the sun is shining? I guess not. We will certainly be camping on the doorstep in September. Everyone will need support during that time, but right now we need to move across state. Teary times for Mom. This graduation. Necessary. Healthy tears.

I hope all your transitions are smooth and tearless.

Prayerfully,

Jan

THE TRANSFORMED CELL

Hilary update

Friday, 08 August 2003

This is a good day. Hilary is feeling very well. The radiation is fast, smooth, and painless. We are now at clinic waiting for someone to remove the sutures from the brain biopsy. It is 3:00 P.M. and we got here around noon.

I finished reading *The Transformed Cell* by Steven Rosenberg. Great book. It is about Dr. Rosenberg's quest to use immunotherapy to stimulate the body's own defenses to fight and even to defeat cancer. He started his research in 1968 and according to Dr. Maziars, Dr. Rosenberg should receive a Nobel Prize for his work in immunotherapy. I found it fascinating! I remember Dad telling me as Mom was dying of her breast cancer that someday scientists and doctors would find a way to remove a few cells, educate them, return them to the body, and those cells would kill the cancer. This is exactly what Dr. Rosenberg is trying to do.

It is now 3:45 P.M., and I've visited on the phone, and I am now using this computer for e-mail. I'm so glad we have these tools of communication during a time of waiting. I probably won't write again for a long while. No news is a status quo situation. I'll write again when we have a plan of action or we receive any new information on Hilary's battle with leukemia.

Can you feel our prayers of blessing for your lives? We can certainly feel your prayers! They are just as real as the warmth of sunshine on

a spring day. Thank you for being diligent in prayer. Our God is an
awesome God!

> Love,
>
> Jan

QUESTIONS ABOUT ANGELS

Hilary update
Saturday, 23 August 2003

Again, I've had many people asking about Hilary, so I thought I'd
send a quick update. Hilary is doing very well! She finished her radiation
and steroids on Tuesday. The radiation has caused her to lose her hair
again and the steroids caused her to have some skin problems, but both
of those side effects are easy to live with. She is busy planning some trips
with her sisters to visit Aunt Peggy and Eagle Valley. She is also planning
to work at the Reserve for a few days during the golf tournament.
Sounds like a normal life, doesn't it? I'm praying that the weekly blood
tests won't show any movement of our enemy so this "normal" life can
go along as intended. I really think the enemy is gone, so Hilary can
complete everything.

I had a great trip to California. Meeting Peggy's friends was like a
family reunion where a person gets to meet unknown cousins. They
were wonderful, loving people! I've been pondering angels and one of
Peggy's friends shared a book about angels with me. I think that was
a God-thing. I haven't had time to read it yet, but I hope the book
answers some of my questions. If you have some insights about angels,
let me know.

These are my questions:

I know that angels are messengers for God, but do they think for
themselves? Demons are angels who have decided to not follow God,
right? So, angels must think if they are going to decide rather to follow

God or not, right? Do they have other decisions? Are they advocates for us or is their main job to point us toward God? Maybe being an advocate is the job of the saints in heaven. Are saints another name for spirit guides? Do angels know the future? Did Hilary's guardian angel know she had leukemia or did her angel just know she was sick? Do angels carry our prayers and messages to God or do they pray with us to God?

While I was pondering angels, I had a cartoon run through my head. Here it is: There are two people with their guardian angels by their sides. One person is in sunshine because he knows "the Light of the World" and his guardian angel is walking directly beside him. The other person is in the dark shadow and his guardian angel has to keep moving back and forth from the sunshine to the shadow in order to see the path well enough to protect his charge.

I thought this was an interesting image. Then I thought if our guardian angels are doing their job, why would anything bad happen? That brought to mind something Mark Lawer said to Tabitha during the last visit at the hospital. Tabitha was just diagnosed with AML the first of July, and Mark had had a transplant last July. They are both strong Christians and Mark said, "I could say that I'm sorry you have leukemia, but I'm also excited. Even though you are starting through this awful valley, I'm excited about what you are going to learn about Jesus. You will meet him with a closeness that you can't find anyplace else." Maybe that's the answer to the question of why we have suffering.

Enough questions. Hilary is well, my school is starting, life is normal. Wonderful! I hope all your lives are normal!

Love,

Jan

GIFTS

Hilary update
20 September 2003

Good morning, everyone. I've tried to write this letter two different times and I just can't get it finished. Maybe my hesitation to write is because I don't like the idea of this second transplant. If I don't tell anyone, it won't happen. Do you think that works?

Last Tuesday, Dr. Fleming and Hilary decided upon October 13 for the beginning of the transplant. Hilary has already started all the tests (hundreds of them, I swear) last week. She is amazing. She is like the WWII veterans Dad has talked about. He tells the story of preparing for his first battle, when the real veterans, who have already seen many battles, came marching in with their attitude of "if there is a bullet for me, there is nothing I can do to stop it, but if I'm supposed to survive, there is nothing that can hurt me." Their guns were packed on their shoulders like our ranchers pack their shovels during irrigation.

Hilary is eager to get started so she can be finished and move on into healing and new growth. She is using the cord blood out of Germany. The broadly matched person from England didn't work out. At first he or she was on vacation and they couldn't find him or her. Then for some reason, this person was unable to be a donor at this time. I pondered of all the possible reasons why someone would remove their name from the list: pregnancy, illness, only did this for a friend and doesn't want to help a stranger, crisis in their own lives and can't add another event, etc., so I wouldn't be so angry about them refusing their stem cells. I know some friends in La Grande are trying to organize a bone marrow drive. Since Hilary can't wait any longer, will this stop those plans? I hope not. Who knows what a drive might produce for another needy person.

Has your mind ever acted like a sieve? You just can't seem to keep any thought in place. Has your mind rumbled around like a truck on a broken road? I've discovered that writing helps me to sort my thoughts and smooth the road. So for those of you who don't like to read my mind-mumbles, please delete now.

I read a devotional a couple of weeks ago about gifts. A lady's house was destroyed by a fire, and when a friend asked if she was able to save anything, her response was, "I only saved what I gave away."

Gifts! I've received many gifts, but two gifts this September are exceptional. First, Doris and her family canned our winter's supply of green beans and tomatoes. What a gift of time! At first I said, "No, that is too much for anyone to do for me." Then Peggy and Tony told me to just say, "Thank you," and accept. Why are some gifts hard to accept?

Then, a former student came to see me during our school's open house. She is now high-school age and away from her mom (Mom is in prison), drug-free for ten months, attending a Christian school in town (as a way to remove herself from her former drug friends), and seems normal! My Richland Methodist Church had prayed for her all during the year she was in my class, and I prayed for her many times thereafter when she came to mind. Even though I prayed for her, I didn't believe God would heal her life. I had put her into the box of lost causes. This was a great lesson in prayer. The thought of "just believe and it will happen" takes the power away from God. It gives us the impression that we are in control. Prayer is our recognition of who God is, not a wish list of what we want. Anyway, it was awesome to see her and pray for her again.

Seeing her has renewed my resolve to pray for my students even more and I'm asking you to join me. I have the same class as last year, because I looped with them to the fourth grade. So, I still have my two boys who need a life change. They need to learn self-control, take responsibility for actions, and develop an attitude of caring for themselves and others. I still have my students whose minds need to be opened to learning. They try so hard and their minds are also sieve-like. Their brains can't seem to hold any memory or understanding. Then I have some students whose minds work extremely well; how do I challenge them into thinking beyond the average?

When I pray for myself and my family, my prayer is basically for our happiness. I thought of the quote from Jesus when he said, I came that they may have life, and have it abundantly. What is abundant life? Isn't it happiness and joy? Doesn't that mean that Hilary will have abundant life? That is certainly my prayer. But my vision of abundant life might be different from God's. So, I went looking for this Scripture, and Jesus said, "The thief comes only in order to steal, kill, and destroy, I have come in order that you might have life—life in all its fullness. I am the good shepherd, who is willing to die for the sheep." John 10:10&11 (TEV) Abundant life is a gift that came when Jesus gave away his life.

So what makes an awesome gift? I've decided that unexpected prayerful gifts are what make gifts awesome. Can I do that? Can I be like cousin Elizabeth who shared her home with pregnant Mary? Can I give my last coin like the widow? Am I like the people in James who ignore needs and say, "I'll pray for you?" I've got a lot more to ponder in my sieve-like mind. I do know that you are gifts to me. I covet your prayers and thank you for taking time to include my concerns in your visits with our God. Please know that I'm praying that you have an "abundant life"!

Love,

Jan

Chapter 10

Peekaboo Drive

Hilary update
Friday, 10 October 2003

Life never goes as planned! Today is Friday the 10th. I'd told everyone good-bye—my class, work partners, church family—moved the dog food to Dad's house, moved the mail and newspaper to Portland, etc., then when I got home tonight, I had a message from Hilary to call as soon as I got in.

The cord blood arrived today, and when they began testing it, it tested positive for the virus Provo. Of course, they are not going to start a transplant process until more testing is complete and much discussion has taken place. Dr. Fleming left Hilary a message on her phone that he thought everything would only be postponed for a week. Hilary thinks that this process will probably take up to three weeks. Nothing moves quickly when testing and discussion are required.

Hilary got her central line in just minutes before the phone call came to wait. Wouldn't you know! Hilary always itches from the tape they use to protect the IV line. In the past, this tape has literally torn Hilary's skin. "Oh, well, I won't have to get poked," was Hilary's response.

Since I've last written, Hilary has had two chemo treatments in the spinal fluid to assure the spot in the brain is truly dead. (Chemo doesn't pass across the blood brain barrier, so they used the spinal fluid.)

The positron emission tomography (PET) scan didn't see any active cells, but the MRI had shown a shadow. The radiation shrank the tumor considerably but didn't melt it completely away. They wanted to make sure that no cells were hiding in that scar tissue. Hilary is also using an alternative program, Nambudripad Allergy Elimination Technique (NAET) energy work, to protect her from chemo side effects. The NAET energy work is to help strengthen her body. When Hilary asked Dr. Fleming about doing this program his response was, "As long as they don't poke, or give you unusual things to eat, go for it." Now Hilary has at least one more week to continue to prepare her body for treatment.

Because I'm here in this quiet house by myself, I have been fighting sadness. Is it hormones? Is it stress? I just know that I'm not sleeping well and tears are always close by. I haven't been able to sing, because my throat tightens. I feel tense and cranky. Then on Wednesday morning, my devotional encouraged me to read Psalms 42 and 43. These words are repeated three times: "Why am I so sad? Why am I so troubled? I will put my hope in God, and once again I will praise him, my savior and my God." Psalms 42:5 & 11 and Psalms 43: 5 (TEV) Why all these sighs? Hope in God! Wow.

That evening I watched the moon play "peekaboo" with me on my drive home. It would show its face, and then hide behind a hill in the canyon. Then it would come out behind that hill, just to hide itself behind the opposite hill. Of course each turn in the canyon road made the moon look like it was moving back and forth yelling, "Peekaboo!" each time it showed itself. Its big, full, yellow face made me laugh.

Sadness, Hope in God, Laughter. What an interesting order of events for one day. Thanks for all the prayers.

Love,

Jan

THOUGHTS

Hilary update
Sunday, 12 October 2003

Today is a blessed day! Because I am not in Portland, I decided to visit the Catholic church in Baker to listen to Jayde, one of my students, play the piano. Jayde invited me last week at school. I arrived early (surprise, I know) and was there for the Rosary. During the part where we are to contemplate the Holy Spirit coming to us, I pondered Pastor Bill's talk about the wonderment of how the Holy Spirit touches some of us during church and others are not touched. He can see one person in tears because the Spirit is moving them, and the person in the next row is sleeping.

Anyway, I decided to look for a touch of the Holy Spirit. During the prayers of the faithful, Father Rob prayed especially for Hilary and all cancer patients. Then during communion, I saw a lady who came up for a special blessing, tears streaming down her face, who did not take communion, and a gentleman behind her guiding her through the maze. I thought, "Wow, I think I just saw a touch of the Holy Spirit."

Then after church, I visited with Nancy until the church was basically empty and the Spanish Mass group was getting things set up for the next service. Father Rob came bustling in and told us to stay for a couple of more minutes, because something wonderful was about to happen. The lady I saw crying in church requested to be baptized, and they were going to do it now. Because she was diagnosed with cancer, Father Rob moved through all the red tape and common practices that cover baptism, first communion, oil of confirmation, and the anointing of the sick, all in a fifteen-minute ceremony. There were ten of us there: the lady's daughter, her daughter's husband, her son, her husband, Nancy, Chuck, Nancy's mom and dad, the lady's sponsor (a friend), and me.

When Father Rob asked for help to lift the baptismal lid, the sponsor said, "I'm not sure that is big enough; I think we need a bathtub!" Everyone laughed. The daughter read the readings, Nancy and I kept smiling at each

141

other, the husband held her glasses, the sponsor whispered explanations when needed, and the lady was obviously touched. We all applauded at the conclusion and I'm sure I heard heaven itself join in the cheer.

When the ceremony ended, the husband stated, "I've been praying for this day," and three other hands lifted in agreement. When the lady went around hugging everyone, I thanked her for letting me be a part of such a special day. What a treat to see the Holy Spirit at work. I wish I could tell her how glad I was that she chose Jesus to be with her while she walks through the valley of the shadow of death. I pray that she continues to feel His rod and staff during the darkest times. I pray that her roots will travel deep into the soil of faith so the evil one cannot pluck her into doubt and confusion.

I think she met this Jesus who stops his walk across the water to get into her lifeboat because she is scared. Maybe she saw a glimmer of how much Jesus loves her. If death-giving cancer can allow us to meet life-giving Jesus, then there is a purpose for this terrible disease. Wow! What a blessed day! What a joyous time!

Well, now that I'm finished, go ahead and forward this to anyone who would understand such a wonderful event, who would be blessed by reading about it, who has also seen the work of the Holy Spirit or would like to know that our God is alive and working in people's lives. Wow. What a day!

Love,

Jan

COLD VIRUS

Hilary update
25 October 2003

This update should have been written last Tuesday evening, but school, driving, and the World Series seemed to have taken all my time. Thus, here is Tuesday's update coming to you from a Saturday morning time slot.

Hilary will begin treatment on November 3, using the cord blood from Germany. It will replace Gabrielle's immune system with a brand-new German immune system that will recognize the evil enemy leukemia. Thank you for all your prayers that this process will be smooth and peaceful and will bring complete healing! We always wonder why things happen in a certain order. Well, Hilary came down with a cold on October 14. I think it was a very good thing the virus in the cord blood made everyone wait for a couple of weeks. The thought of Hilary starting chemo on the 13th, then trying to fight a cold with a dying immune system on the 14th is beyond scary.

As it is, Hilary still has a terribly stuffed nose and is taking antibiotics. I wish she weren't going into this procedure weakened, but I know nothing of the future. I remind myself, "Remember, God loves this girl more than you and he is in control."

On Tuesday, Hilary will have a bone marrow biopsy to check the health of her blood. I'm sure everything will be clean!

I've been told to read Exodus 23:20–33 twice in the last couple of months. So now I'm pondering what God means when he says, "Little by little," and "an angel to precede you." Maybe all God really wants is prayer and communion? Something else to ponder.

I thank you for your prayers. I have felt joyful since my last e-mail and I know your prayers are part of that. Thank you.

Love,
Jan

Sinus

Hilary update
04 November 2003

Good afternoon. I wrote a wonderfully witty letter this morning, then in the process of spell check, an error came on the screen and it got deleted. Something has to be wrong with the apartment computer. Now I am making another attempt at e-mail, and Kris, Hilary's nurse, just came in to tell me we have ten to fifteen minutes before Hilary's eye, ear, and nose doctor takes a look. We have waited all morning for this test. I told Kris, Hilary, and Tony not to leave without me, but I'd write until a transport came. (I've learned that ten to fifteen minutes in this hospital can turn out to be two hours. Patience is a very good virtue to possess at hospitals.)

I will now give you a summarized version of this morning's letter: Hilary came in last night as scheduled. She is in room 13, the same room she had the transplant in last year. Home, sweet home. She has not started radiation because she is still fighting some sinus stuff from the cold she caught in October. Thus, she had a CAT scan of her sinus and of her lungs last night. Today she is having a sinus suction. She had a nasal wash last night and they are culturing the stuff. (Don't you wish you worked in a lab? You get to play with a lot of gross stuff.) I truly hope this sinus problem is just bacteria or a virus and not our evil enemy. Tony said that it shouldn't be because of where the blood and sinus are connected. I hope Tony is right. No doctor has mentioned that this stuffed sinus could be the enemy. My mind just seems to think about the worst possible problem. Sometimes this method of thinking is a good coping technique because you can problem-solve. Not true to this situation. Forgive me. Where is my faith?

Hilary informed us that she did not want us discussing who got to stay with her at 11:00 at night, and then to say, "You decide, Hilary." (I don't remember ever saying, "You decide, Hilary. Who do you want to stay with you?") We are to make that decision before entering the hospital, or at least not while in her room. So, Irene took Sunday and Monday nights because she doesn't work on Monday and Tuesday. Gabrielle took Wednesday and Friday because she doesn't have classes on Thursday and Saturday. I get Tuesday, Thursday, and Saturday. Then when Elizabeth comes, I'll give her my Saturday time slot. Wouldn't you love to be so popular that people fight over who can stay with you?

Of course, OHSU and Hilary will see Tony and me during the daylight hours every day.

Well, my ten minutes are up, and I'm going to spell check this letter before the nurse comes. Love to all of you. Hope you get this.

Love,

Jan

P.S. I didn't get the spell check finished. OHSU kept true to their ten to fifteen minutes. Thus, I saved this as a draft, and now it is Tuesday morning. The eye, ear, nose man was very nice. Tony and I got to watch a TV screen showing the scope's picture of Hilary's nose. Fascinating. Her nose was clear, but when he looked at the CAT scan, which we also got to see, Hilary's left sinus was full of junk. The draining area from that sinus is really small and so that is probably why it filled up. Anyway, after discussion with his boss and with Dr. Leis, Hilary is taking antibiotics for two weeks, plus two nasal sprays. She gets to come back home on Wednesday and will probably go back on Sunday. They are postponing the transplant one more week, and so the second week of antibiotics will be the first week of treatment.

Hilary will still have warrior cells to fight the sinus problem during the first week of treatment. Of course, the staff will check to see if the antibiotics are doing their job before starting. They also took a culture of this sinus problem, so we should know within three days the name of this junk.

It is now 7:00 A.M. and the overcast sky looks the same as dawn at home. It's no wonder people in Portland don't start moving until later. I'm going to try Curves, which is only a mile from the apartment. It opens at 6:45 or 7:00 A.M. Baker City's Curves opens at 5:30. Early here means a totally different time than early in Eastern Oregon.

Yesterday, Hilary, Irene, and I read *In the Year of the Boar and Jackie Robinson* while Tony studied pre-nursing classes. It is one of the novels my fourth-grade class will read. Bandit, the main character in the book, moved from China to New York City. My location change is minor

145

compared to Bandit's but I do feel a cultural difference from Eastern Oregon to Western Oregon. We might speak the same language, but some of our words have different pictures. For example, "early."

Well, I need to go so we can get to the hospital. May all our words produce grand pictures of love, kindness, and truth.

Love,
Jan

P.P.S. I haven't sent this yet. I was afraid of the computer at the apartment, so I saved it as a draft again. We've seen some friends that had transplants last year and they are doing great. Lisa from the clinic walked over during her lunch break to bring Hilary an angel plaque. There are some good things—or I should say, some very good people—who really care about us here. Very special. I'm sending this now.

Love,
Jan

FIRST RADIATION DAY

Hilary update
12 November 2003

Hilary started her full-body radiation today. She will have ten-minute treatments every morning and afternoon for four days. They are giving her 23 megavolts (MV) energy with 175 cbyx2, 300 per day. I asked the therapist for those numbers on the screen because I thought Wade would like to know, even if they don't mean anything to me. Maybe he will explain them to me. Than again, maybe he shouldn't. Oblivion is a wonderful tool to ward off worries.

Hilary sits in a soft black chair with her knees drawn to her chest. She gets to listen to music, while she sits really still. Today she said she fell asleep during the treatment. They put a plexus glass between her and the machine. Apparently, the glass distributes the rays more evenly. After half the time, they flip her around. As I watched the rotation, I could smell something like a summer rain shower. It was ozone in the room. The door between the therapist's desk and the radiation room is at least one foot thick. I think it is the door that proves this treatment is dangerous. The radiation therapist has about six monitors in front of her. I watched the monitor showing Hilary quietly sitting in the black chair. I'm glad my job requires looking at children's faces. Watching those monitors would not only be overwhelming, but not fun.

I did notice a wonderful large plate of cookies close to the station. I asked if it was for a staff's birthday celebration. They were from a patient who'd had his last day of radiation. Wasn't that a nice thing to do? Isn't that like a birthday celebration? Because of OHSU's skills with this powerful energy, this cookie person will be able to celebrate more birthdays. After Hilary is finished with radiation, she will have chemo for two days, have a day off, and then the stem cell transplant will be on the next day. The nurse told Hilary last night that the cord blood's blood type was B negative. Hilary said, "I like being A negative." It was one of the first times that Hilary has expressed some disappointment or hesitation in this whole event. Irene and I are talkers. But Tony, Hilary, Gabrielle, and Elizabeth are not. When they say something, we need to grip it tight.

Rosemary came yesterday afternoon to do some yoga with us. It was very relaxing. She said she will try to come at least twice a week. Of course, everything is contingent upon Hilary's reactions to treatments.

Mark came by to visit this morning. Ryan and Heidi also came to visit Hilary before they joined Gabrielle and Todd for Ryan's birthday dinner, and then Father Rob came to visit this afternoon. Father Rob from Baker City anointed Hilary with oil and laid hands upon her. Our extended, supportive Christian family is absolutely awesome. You are all part of that family. You are awesome.

Love,

Jan

SECOND RADIATION DAY

Hilary update, Tuesday and Wednesday
Thursday, 13 November 2003

The second day of radiation is almost finished. There is now no turning back. Hilary is doing very well with it. She has a thickening of her saliva and that is all.

Now, a couple of stories about funny stuff in hospital life. I'll start with the bed story.

When we got here on Sunday, they didn't have an extra bed for the overnight-caretaking family member. Elizabeth got a wonderful leather recliner to sleep in. Then, last night (Irene's night), we asked again for a bed and around 11:00 P.M. they brought one. Because the scales on Hilary's bed didn't work, they gave Irene Hilary's bed and Hilary has the new bed with the working scale. Unfortunately, the new bed's control didn't work, so Hilary couldn't adjust her bed up and down, control the light, or call the nurse with a call button. Then at 4:00 A.M., the nurse tried to weigh Hilary using the bed scale, and Hilary weighed 400 pounds. Everyone knows that isn't correct, so Hilary still had to get out of bed to stand on the scale next to the nurses' station. They are waiting now for a bed technician to find out why the bed's control is not working. Hilary and I will trade beds tonight if this new bed with the working scale (ha, ha) isn't fixed.

Second, Hilary was walking the halls when the fire alarm went off. The doors in the middle of the hall closed and she was on the wrong side to get to her room. She continued her walk in the now-shortened hall, until her nurse came and found her. During a fire alarm, all the patients are supposed to be in their rooms. Hilary had escaped...ha, ha.

Wednesday: Today is more of the same. Hilary and I figured that thirty laps in the hall would make a mile. The technician fixed the bed. No other real news. Boring, as always, is a great place to be.

Let me tell you about some of the patients here. First is Mike. He's twenty-two years old. He is married and has the cutest little boy, about a year old, who is just learning to walk. We met him a week ago on our second false start of this transplant. We met his mom first. It was about 7:30 in the evening when Hilary and I were going to walk on the sky bridge and I made a quick detour into the bathroom while Hilary collected an elevator. Hilary kept hitting the elevator button and when the doors opened, she would apologize, embarrassed because I wasn't out of the bathroom yet. Then she would hit the elevator button again, expecting me to be there before the next elevator arrived. Well, after three elevator stops, she came to save me from the bathroom. I was talking with Mike's mom. I could tell the woman needed to visit.

Apparently, Mike has AML and was very hesitant to get a transplant. He received one day of radiation and told them to wait. A patient can still stop the process after one day of radiation, but after the second day of radiation a patient is too far on the diving board to turn around.

Mike's mom visited with Mike's wife four times during the day and shed many tears of fear that Mike was going to refuse this procedure. She knew with Mike's one relapse of AML, this was the next logical solution for a possible cure. Mike did proceed with a radiation treatment in the afternoon. We asked his mom if Mike would like some visitors. So, when Hilary and I got back from our walk, we visited with Mike. He didn't respond to us. He seemed very depressed. He mentioned that he felt pressured into this ordeal. We said that we'd pray for him, and his mom said their pastor was coming sometime this week. The next day before we left for home, we visited again and shared Mark's message of "We could say 'sorry about the awful valley you are beginning,' but there is something very exciting about how your relationship with Jesus will grow." I know I didn't say it as well as when Mark visited with Tabitha, but I prayed for him to know the reason and purpose for suffering. When Mike got his transplant yesterday, he told us that his attitude was better and thanked us for our visit. This made me feel as if we had some purpose for being here.

Then there is another Mike down the hall who is reading *The Purpose Driven Life* by Rick Warren. Mike and his wife are wonderful Christians. He is finished with his transplant and is traveling home tomorrow.

There is also a David, who has diabetes and is experiencing a GVH problem from a transplant last May. He seems self-assured and confident. Great to see but I feel nervous about this GVH.

These are amazing people who are swimming in this pond called cancer. Some are confident, some are worried, some are angry, and some are planting their roots deep into their baptismal water of life. All are amazing.

Love you bunches,

Jan

P.S. Thursday morning: I didn't get this sent earlier. Just thought I'd let you know that Mike and Gail down the hall brought Hilary a copy of the book, *The Purpose Driven Life*. It was such a nice surprise gift. Twenty-two-year-old Mike came to visit Hilary in her room and had a great smile on his face. Tony and I visited with Jerry and Marie at the VA hospital. It was such a nice reunion with my Tillamook family. The last time we saw Jerry and Marie was at our wedding twenty-five years ago. It is amazing how easy it is to visit when we are family in Christ.

Thanks for your prayers for Hilary, and now you have a few more names to add to the list.

Love you bunches,

Jan

P.P.S. The bed still doesn't work.

SATURDAY MORNING HILARY UPDATE

Hilary update
15 November 2003

Oh, boy, here we go. Hilary started Cytoxan and Atgam yesterday. She seems to do fine with the Cytoxan, which continues decreasing her white blood cells. But after the Atgan, which is an immune suppressant made from a protein from horse-blood products, she became extremely nauseated and a puffy, red hive-looking rash crossed her face. Then she started running a temperature. At midnight they took a chest x-ray, took blood cultures, and a urine culture. They were looking for a bacterium that might cause these side effects. I think the rash and temperature are from the Atgam. She's supposed to receive Cytoxan and Atgam again today, plus start Tacrolimus, another immunosuppressive drug. I hope they reconsider Hilary's plan. I don't think this is a good start! She is only 96 pounds. She doesn't have any reserves. She wasn't supposed to react to the Atgam like this. Yuk! I'm numb.

I flipped a coin with Gabrielle and I won the toss to stay at the hospital. I need to stretch a little, so here I am in a bright room typing to you. I'll now go back to Hilary's dim room and watch her sleep. They try to keep Hilary very comfortable, which means sleep. Drugs, they kill and they heal. Can you imagine putting something from a horse inside of you? No wonder Hilary's body went ballistic. I would, too! Talk to you later.

Love,
Jan

Love, Jan

SATURDAY AFTERNOON

Hilary update
Saturday, 15 November 2003

Things are better. Thought I'd drop a line after my awful e-mail this morning. I needed to complain. When I got back to the room I called to cancel Linda and Ron's visit. Linda prayed for all of us over the phone. What a wonderment is the strength and comfort provided by a faithful believer's prayer. As I leaned over my sleeping Hilary, praying for a better day, repeating some of Linda's phrases, I thought of childbirth. This process of preparing for a new immune system is somewhat like childbirth. No fun, but necessary if new life is to begin. That got me thinking about the joy of a new baby and I felt again that hope of healing.

When Carol, one of the nurse practitioners, came to visit today, she told Hilary they would come to visit her on next year's birthday. They would just shut down OHSU and come celebrate. (Hilary and Gabe's twentieth birthday is the 22nd of November; the transplant last year was on the 21st, and this year's transplant will be on the 17th.) I'm already planning a fantastic twenty-first birthday party! You're all invited.

Love,
Jan

LOST DAY

Hilary update
Sunday, 16 November 2003

You would find it hard to believe the difference between our laughing, card-playing girl on Thursday evening and the curled up child on Friday evening. Dell came to the hospital planning to drive Tony to Eastern Oregon for Treasure Valley's pre-nursing test. I was planning to drive Tony, but when I looked at our coiled daughter, I couldn't think of leaving. Yet, I was concerned for Tony. He had too much packed into one day, with class and travel, so having a driver would ease the load a little. Friday's class on anatomy and physiology finished at 8:00 P.M. Then Tony and I were planning to drive all night to get to Ontario on Saturday morning. With his worrying about Hilary, he is just running on adrenalin, and I'm passing my driving duties to Dell.

When Hilary started running a temperature, with the hive-looking rash on her face, I couldn't leave. Even though the nurses were taking Hilary's vitals every fifteen minutes, I was watching for any changes during those other fourteen minutes. I was afraid the swelling rash would move to the throat. I had gotten myself into quite a worrying state. Then Tony refused Dell's kindness and drove by himself.

Hilary's temperature went to 101.5 after the infusion had finished and the nurses were back into the routine of checking vitals every four hours. So, I would take her temperature every half hour, just to keep tabs. I'm glad there is a thermometer on Hilary's wall. At 11:30 P.M., I asked the nurse if Hilary could have some Tylenol. "Absolutely," was the answer. They had taken some blood cultures earlier because of this temperature. Then the nurse called the night doctor, who came to check Hilary about midnight. I pointed out the receding rash left on Hilary's chin and gave him a summary of the evening's events, because Hilary was not really explaining things well (the Benadryl really makes Hilary sleepy). So, the doctor ordered a chest x-ray and a culture of Hilary's urine. I slept the night on top of the covers, fully dressed with my shoes ready to put on. I felt that Hilary's rash, temperature, vomiting, and chills were all side effects of that "horse stuff." I wondered if Hilary had made a smart decision about doing this transplant.

Then today, they gave her more pre-meds, and slowed down the infusion from four hours to over five hours. Hilary seemed to tolerate it very well. No rash, no vomiting, no temperature, no curling body. OHSU doesn't know about Linda's prayer, Dell's prayer, Tony's prayer, and Dad's prayer; plus I know Julie went back to the school-board convention and told all of Pine Eagle School Board that I wouldn't let them in to see Hilary because she wasn't doing well, and they all prayed for her. Tom Crane, the superintendent and principal, came to see Hilary today and he knew Hilary wasn't doing well.

He was concerned whether her attitude was still good. Her attitude is wonderful. But she can't remember yesterday. When I mentioned Irene's work schedule, Hilary said yesterday's schedule. She thought I had visited Holly this morning and I visited Holly yesterday morning.

She said, "But you ran to the apartment this morning."

"No honey," I said, "I did that yesterday."

Maybe it is a good thing she can't remember yesterday afternoon, but then again, that's another confirmation that my big concern was valid.

She has to take this "horse stuff" (Atgam) one more day. Then next week she has three days of Methotrexate, which is known to cause those awful mouth sores.

You can tell I'm tired. I sure ramble a lot when I get tired. I'm at the apartment with Irene, and Gabrielle is spending the night with Hilary. Thank you, thank you, thank you again for everything you do. Thank you, thank you, thank you (I don't think I could thank you enough).

Jan

NEW BIRTHDAY

Hilary update, day 0, evening
Monday, 17 November 2003

A new birthday. When I got to the hospital this morning, Hilary informed me that she didn't sleep well last night. Her stomach hurt. Gabe asked if she was nervous. Hilary shrugged and responded, "I don't think so." The stem cells were to arrive around 11:00 A.M. but the nurse said to expect them around noon. Hilary showered at 11:30, and as soon as the shower was finished nausea became "the boss." Hilary said Lisa, her naturopath, was coming as soon as she could. Lisa treated Hilary with NAET for a couple of weeks preparing for this transplant. NAET is an alternative health program dealing with frequencies and body energy. Please look it up on the Internet for more information. Lisa is an anesthesiologist by trade and works with NAET part-time.

When the cells showed up around 2:00 P.M. and Lisa walked into the room seconds before they started infusion, I thought, "Is this a God-thing? The timing is more than coincidence." Hilary had asked the doctors last week about Lisa working with her and the blood before transfusion and after some questions, they said, "Fine." I think Lisa was surprised at their consent but as Nurse Carol said to me, "You know, people think that they must choose between traditional medicine and alternative medicine. These two ideas should be a marriage, not a choice." Thus, the doctors allowed Lisa to test frequencies and then do some work before they started the infusion.

During infusion (which lasted over an hour), Lisa, Carol, Nurse David, and I never left the room. Dr. Marrow popped in many times. I think Hilary was the first adult patient to ever receive stem cells from a cord blood at OHSU. David said the blood looked different from that of an adult donor. Hilary's vital signs stayed very normal. She sat in a chair with a bucket, in case her stomach complained, and watched all of us watching her. Lisa did circles on Hilary's body gates. David kept moving between the monitor, recording vitals and the pole holding the blood bag. Carol watched the monitor and any flushing or other ill symptoms from Hilary (there were none), and I held the bucket when necessary. The stem cells are preserved in dimethyl sulfoxide (DMSO) before freezing, and the DMSO makes people sick. Hilary smells like sweet garlic from the DMSO. I thought of Grandpa Joe, who bought DMSO from the vet for his arthritis.

Dr. Marrow brought Hilary a copy of *Glamour* magazine, which had an article from one of his patients who has chronic myelogenous leukemia (CML). She was a writer before her cancer fight and is now journaling about her cancer experiences in this magazine. She will be in Portland during December, and Dr. Marrow wants Hilary to meet her.

When I looked at the magazine, it shows the same bed Gabrielle used on the fourteenth floor for her apheresis donation. Take a look at page 144 of the December (2003) issue. Apparently, Dr. Marrow has all the issues of her journal sitting beside his medical books.

Then, I met a new patient who just moved in today and who has been praying for Hilary since the last weekend. They are from The Dalles. When Tony drove home last Friday night he was pulled over by a police officer for not having a light over the license plate. While Tony was looking for his driver's license, the officer noticed Hilary and Gabe's school picture for basketball. As they were talking, Tony mentioned that Hilary was at OHSU. Well, the officer's very good friend, Willie, was going to OHSU for a stem cell transplant soon. The police officer asked if he could he pray for Hilary. So, the officer, Willy, and his wife Rhonda have been praying for Hilary before they even met her.

Rhonda is a Christian musician who just cut a CD, and she gave us a copy. Her CDs are helping to pay for medical costs. Now you can pray for Willie and check out Rhonda's website. It is www.rhondafunk. com. I haven't checked it out yet, but her CD is pretty nice.

Then Gabe, Todd, Irene, and Irene's friend Robert, and I finished the day's celebration with Chinese food, while Hilary held her barf bucket and smiled at some of the stories. Tony called twice while in Richland, sick with an awful cold. I'm so sorry he has a cold and will not be able to visit for probably two weeks. This mean old virus has made him an outcast. I'm sure it is caused from lack of sleep and stress. It is just terrible. I'm glad I stayed in Portland Friday night instead of driving him home, or I would have been an outcast, too. Tony is handling this isolation much better than I would have. I would be so vocal!

Even though there are some parts of this day that are yucky, I am amazed by the timing of Lisa and the stem cells, meeting a total stranger who has been praying for Hilary, and feeling the support of your prayers. Wow, what a birthday!

Love,
Jan

FLOOR MATES

Hilary update, Tuesday, 1:00 A.M.
Tuesday, 18 November 2003

I just read last night's update and I see many mistakes. I can tell my tired, sieve-like mind is really not working. You are all so kind to not make fun of me and my writing. At least you don't make fun of me to my face. Thank you.

Debbie brought in a copy of Teisha's cover for her new CD of Amelia. We have it taped to the hospital wall. Apparently, Amelia has earned some excellent reviews. I love Teisha's voice! I think she will be sending an e-mail about her first experience with chemo. I do know she is in San Francisco right now, singing with her band. Her cancer is not slowing her down much. She is amazing.

When Gabe and I got here around 9:00 A.M., Hilary looked really good. Then the stomach had to do its thing, and so she is now sleeping again. The anti-nausea medicine really puts her to sleep. I don't care. She might as well sleep through this time of her life. I don't think there is anything she would like to remember. Today, they give her the Methotrexate, which may cause mouth sores. Yuk.

We saw Tabitha in the parking lot elevator today. She will be coming in for her transplant next Monday. This floor is becoming full of Christians. I think we ought to start our own Bible study. So, you now have two more names added to your list: Willie and Tabitha. Plus, add Katie from down the hall to your list. She has lymphoma, where the T-cells are affected. Her transplant is just buying her time in hope that something better will come about before her evil cancer shows back up. I think everyone else is here for a cure, where Katie is in here for a delay.

Katie and Hilary had their radiation back-to-back. So, many days I would wheel Katie back to the floor instead of having her wait for transport. Last Sunday she gave Hilary a beautiful ceramic angel. She told Hilary the angel wanted to stay with her. Now the angel is sitting next to the CD player. Hilary has received so many gifts from people who are in the same pond as she. Everyone seems so concerned for everybody else. Such love!

Oh my, I've been here way too long. Hilary just came looking for me. Got to go. Love you bunches. Thanks for being my listening ear.

Love,

Jan

LIPIDS

Hilary update, day 2
Wednesday, 19 November 2003

Food is a big job! Yesterday, I would read a couple of pages, Hilary would take two bites and two sips, and then I would read some more. She only kept in the body one-half cup of soup. Every time she had to take her antibiotic, which was four times a day, the food would come back up. Now she has had two days with very few calories. Today they changed every pill but one to intravenous. And tonight they plan to give her the "white food in the bottle" (I think it is called lipids) through those lifesaving ports in her chest. Her throat is sore. I was praying the mouth sores, mucositis, would not be bad this time, but a sore throat isn't a good start.

Once God set our bodies into a pattern, he hasn't changed that pattern very often. Sometimes it's hard to accept that our loving God doesn't just take away all this suffering instead of holding our hand through it all. Yet, when Jesus holds our hand, the suffering seems less intense. That's hard to believe, isn't it?

Love,

Jan

Baby Schedule

Hilary update, day 3
Thursday, 20 November 2003

Things are better! No vomiting yesterday (except at 3:00 A.M. this morning) and Hilary was able to retain one-half cup of soup, one cup of chicken broth, one-half cup of yogurt, one-half of a cheese stick, and two cups of root beer (which surprises me that she requested root beer with such a sore throat). She has a baby's schedule: awake for a couple of hours in the morning while slowly eating her soft, minimal breakfast. Then she takes a nap for a couple of hours. When lunch arrives, she's again awake for a couple of hours while drinking her chicken broth. After that, she takes another couple-hour nap. With that kind of schedule, don't you think those baby cells should think this body is where they're supposed to be and say, "What a nice home"?

Yesterday afternoon Rosemary came and did some energy work with Hilary. After the energy work, Hilary requested some yoga. When I got back to the hospital, Hilary seemed much better, more alert and strong. Today, her mouth is red, along with a really red throat. The nurses keep reminding Hilary she can request pain medicine for the sore mouth. Hilary hasn't requested any yet. They work so hard to keep the patients as comfortable as possible. Dr. Marrow said, "The first couple of days were just a bump in the road."

I agree—just a bump in the road—but it's just a little scary when you're up in the air wondering how long you're going to float, and praying the road is still there when you come down. I've almost hit the ditch a few times with bumps on those frozen dirt roads at home. I don't want Hilary to hit a ditch, because then we'd have to get the tractor and pull her out. I don't want to see the tractors they have at OHSU. I think they're all in the ICU unit.

Anyway, today is better!

Love, Jan

Willie's friends at The Dalles are going to have a benefit football game this weekend between the police and Les Schwab. (Willie works for Les Schwab and his great friend, whom Tony met, is a police officer.) They're calling it "The Pig Bowl." Of course, Willie is here and won't be able to see this game. This reminded me of all the stuff you guys did for Hilary: Over the Hill for Hilary, spaghetti feed with a pie auction, silent auction with soup and entertainment. Our communities are really awesome. You are really awesome! Thank you for loving us! Thank you for praying for us!

Love,
Jan

PCA

Hilary update, day 4 (fwd)
Friday, 21 November 2003

Nurse Karen got Hilary a new pole yesterday. She stole it from 5A. It is the second-best pole for holding pumps, etc., and when the people on 5A said, "Hey, where are you taking that pole?" and Karen told them it was for Hilary, taking the pole became all right. I guess there is one advantage to being here so much. Everyone knows you. Then, this morning they added a patient-controlled analgesia (PCA) to Hilary's pole.

Hilary starting asking for some pain relief last night for her mouth and throat. When the nurse asked her to rate her pain between one and ten, Hilary said eight. That is the first time I've heard Hilary say a number above five. She received one pain med, and that caused her to vomit. Then she received another, which held off the pain for a couple of hours. I had thought PCA meant "pain control apparatus," but it's really "patient-controlled analgesia." Hilary can press a button and self-administer pain drugs to herself every six minutes, if needed.

160

The antifungal IV medication that Hilary is taking is good-old Amphotericin, which we call "shake and bake." I asked Hilary if maybe she could take the pill instead of "shake and bake," but she preferred "shake and bake" over swallowing a pill. Another big message as to how much her throat hurts. Antifungal medicine is really tough stuff. I always thought that bacteria were the worst germs out there, but fungus is one step beyond the wicked bacteria. The antifungal meds are the worst. At least Hilary only has to take Amphotericin three times a week, not every day like last year, which is the difference between fighting an already existing fungus and preventing fungus.

Irene needs to go to work, so I'm closing. Love you all bunches.

Love,

Jan

BIRTHDAY

Hilary update, day 5
Saturday, 22 November 2003

I'm at the apartment and have only ten minutes before I go to the VA hospital for church. OHSU doesn't have a chapel, so people go to the VA hospital for any worship service.

Yesterday, the girls' birthday, was wonderful and miserable. Hilary was miserable. Her mouth sores are yucky! She doesn't talk, but uses facial expressions and hand signals to communicate. I told her she reminded me of Phyllis, and she shook her finger at me, just the way Phyllis would do. Of course, I meant that she was communicating like the way Phyllis does. Hilary and Phyllis are certainly completely different people.

The wonderful parts are: Judith came in the morning to give Hilary a craniosacral therapy treatment. Then, Yen and Amy came to visit. Their visits made this day extra special. And the kitchen sent up a birthday cake, which was really pretty good. We all had a piece except one of the birthday girls. Guess which one? And she wasn't refusing because of a diet issue.

Of course, Tony missed the day because of his cold. He is so strong about this. I get panicked every time I feel a small scratch in my throat. Todd now has a cold, and he missed Gabrielle's birthday, because Gabrielle spent the day with Hilary. Hilary is running a temperature off and on. She has a rash that covers her entire head. Yesterday morning, because of swelling from the rash, her right eye looked as if someone punched her. I worry about throat swelling.

More Benadryl seems to be the answer to control of the rash. They're not too eager to delete medicines in search of a cause. They just want to control the problem. The awfulness of this suffering is that it probably won't quit until Hilary's baby stem cells begin to create the new immune system.

We're looking at a good ten days of this! Ten days. Ten days of this misery while waiting. At least we know there is an end. I think of those people who were in concentration camps. They didn't know when the end would be. Pray that Hilary's courage continues. This is really hard to watch. It must be really, really hard to endure!

I'm beginning to cry. Better close. Thanks for your continued prayers. I'm reading and praying about "why there is suffering" and I know that Jesus refused pain medicine on the cross. Can you believe that? He even experienced great pain on the Mount of Olives because he knew what was ahead of him. He didn't want it. His sweat was like drops of blood while he continued to say, "Not my will, but your will, God." He knows about suffering. Not just suffering of body, but suffering of rejection.

Hilary is supported in every way possible for her suffering. I'm thinking of Thanksgiving and I'm thankful for nausea and pain medicine. I'm thankful for wonderful nurses. I'm thankful for family. I'm thankful for you. And I'm thankful to my friend Jesus, who has held my hand and suffered those awful whippings across his back so that we might be healed. This is just a bump in the road. God is in control of the path. It sure is rough right now.

Jan

No Change

Hilary update, days 7 and 8
Tuesday, 25 November 2003

The baby stem cells are one week old. I hope they are saying, "Yes, what a wonderful place this is. This will be a wonderful home. Everyone is making us feel so welcome." Can't you envision all the cells talking to each other? Hilary had her last shot of Methotrexate last night. This chemo kills the T-cells that cause GVHD. Thus, they use Methotrexate to alleviate some GVH. Today they gave Hilary a shot of leucovorin to prevent the Methotrexate from doing any more harm. I picture the chemo as an acid and today's leucovorin as an antacid. Then, they started some Neupogen to encourage those baby stem cells to grow. Day seven is a good day—the beginning of life, the ending of death. It is amazing what they know about drugs. I think of all those people who were in medical clinical trials, like my nephew Jerome. He died of leukemia, but he was one of those in the early trials that advanced treatment for other patients.

Day 8: You won't receive any new message today. In this case, "no news is good news." Hilary is much better. Not a ton better, but much better. Her mouth sores are still just terrible, but she is certainly taking control. Using the PCA and mouthwash seems to help. The mouthwash is powerful stuff. They make it up special in the pharmacy and it numbs the mouth. Last night, I heard her swish with mouthwash every hour. Today, her lower lip doesn't look as swollen. After she woke from her nap, she told me that she was dreaming of a wonderful sandwich with a nice leaf of lettuce, tomato, olives, and cucumbers. Then she swallowed.

The swallow woke her up…pain. Everyone reminds her that this pain is only temporary. Stay strong. (Hilary is very strong! No complaints from this warrior!)

They moved Katie yesterday to floor 5A. Tom, her husband, is fairly put out. I don't blame him. I think it is because they needed a room for Tabitha, and Katie's counts are coming in. Then Michael told us that he gets to go home tomorrow. Now, I think the reason they moved Katie is because Michael and Tabitha have children who visit often. In fact, I think Austin, Tabitha's five-year-old son, will be staying here with Mom and Dad for the duration of transplant. Tom and Katie both feel disrupted and unimportant. They wonder why this has happened. I can only trust that this hospital is trying to help all their patients the best they can. I also know that Hilary hated being on 5A. 5A is a hospital, where 5C is like a dorm community.

Gail Vaughn, the lady who gave Hilary the book *The Purpose Driven Life*, came to visit Hilary while Mike, her husband, was at clinic. It was so nice to see her. Hilary thrives on visitors. Michael came to play some cards, got a little tired, and climbed right into the extra bed. Joyce, his grandmother, and I visited for probably three hours while Michael and Hilary slept. It surprised me that Michael made himself so comfortable in our room. I'm glad he did.

Then Holly Bandeen and her mom, Irene, came to the barrier doors to let us know that Holly is going home today or tomorrow. Holly has been on the fourteenth floor for at least two weeks. Hilary has been concerned about Holly's health, so I've tried to visit every day in order to give Hilary a report. Holly is such a sweet girl and she is going to have a long road toward healing. Mike, Holly's dad, told me, "If Holly has a good day, I can sleep at night when I go home. If Holly has a bad day, I don't sleep well." Boy, do I know that parental reaction. Please pray for Holly. She has a really long battle, which is not cancer, but a long battle just the same.

Are your prayer calluses big enough yet? I just keep adding to your list.

Later on day 8: I left the computer for a few minutes and another gentleman was typing. His wife is on 5A with a number of complications to cope with before she can have a transplant. It sounded very scary. Her name is Kelly. They have three small kids and this dad seemed a bit "wowed" about everything.

I keep meeting people who need prayer. This place is full of needy people! They share their stories so willingly. It just seems that the people in hospitals recognize the need for prayer. I think we need more monks in the world who make it their career to pray constantly. Until then, it's up to us. Whatever time you devote to your prayer life, this selfish mom appreciates your prayers for us. I know you are praying because I can feel Jesus' presence! Can you feel my prayers for you?

Love,
Jan

Room Decorations

Hilary update, day 9
Wednesday, 26 November 2003

More of the same...boring. Hilary is enduring mouth sores while she waits for engraftment. She has two drugs to help fight GVH and one drug to encourage stem cell growth. I asked Dr. Fleming yesterday about the immune system and the blood brain barrier. He said that Hilary will probably have a few more chemo treatments in her spinal column to mop up any remaining evil cells in her brain. Of course, my brain immediately went to "Why are we doing this? Gabe's immune system did not let any evil cells enter the bone marrow. If Hilary needs more chemo for the brain, then you're not sure this baby immune system is going to eliminate any evil cells in the brain. Why are we doing this?"

Tony said, "Jan, don't go there. We can only go forward. This was Hilary's decision." So now I've said it. I'm done. We can't go back, but

I do wish I had been here two months ago to ask this question. Never mind. This is not my battle with cancer; this is Hilary's battle with cancer. My job is to write e-mails and pray.

Let me tell you about Hilary's room. We've changed a few things since we were here last year. We copied Tabitha's bed arrangement, with the visitor bed directly under the window. That provides an open space for chairs and visitors. Gabe painted a beautiful, 24-by-18-inch, brightly colored picture of many objects. Almost everyone who enters makes a comment about how much they like the picture. I hope Gabe gives it to me. I like it, too. Then Angela, one of Irene's friends, came and created a window-like effect using material. Abbey and Jennifer brought a large balloon of Eeyore, which now flies from one of the closet doors. Of course, Hilary brought the Christmas lights, Grandma's blanket, Petey, and her pillow, just like last year.

I could write a children's book about Hilary's experiences using Petey's viewpoint. Petey is a soft, yellow toy duck that Jamie gave to Hilary. He has certainly been a part of each trip here. Claire, one of Hilary's nurses, always asks Petey to hold the lines as she untangles stuff. All of the staff knows his name. He is an important part of Hilary's room.

Ever since Hilary got the DVD extended version of *Two Towers* for her birthday, Irene made it a goal to get the DVD player working so Hilary could watch it. The day nurses put in a request for a TV maintenance man to come and look at the hookups. When that didn't happen, Irene asked the night nurses. Sweet Emily, our night nurse, had a gentleman up here within half an hour. He looked things over and said, "I'll be right back," and brought in a new video player that would allow us to attach the DVD player. The next customer in room 13 will have a new video player because of Irene's persistence.

It is warm, fuzzy, and comfortable in Hilary's room, thanks to many hands who love her! Have a wonderful, blessed Thanksgiving. Our thankful list includes you. Hope you are feeling extremely blessed.

Love,
Jan

Chapter 10

THANKSGIVING DAY

Hilary update, day 12
Saturday, 29 November 2003

I'm at the apartment, but thought I'd drop a few words before I went to the hospital. We hope everyone had a wonderful Thanksgiving. Our day was similar to last year. The faces were different, but the bald heads looked similar. Irene cooked a delicious turkey, even though OHSU had provided a turkey dinner. We hadn't heard about a floor dinner this year, so we bought enough supplies to feed a lot of people. Then on Tuesday, Leslie sent a flier to everyone about providing a Thanksgiving meal on the floor. Normally they do this dinner the week before Thanksgiving and everyone from the clinic comes over, but last year's coordinator retired. Thus, Leslie went to work asking drug companies to fund a dinner, and had a caterer bring it all in. Irene said, "I've already bought a fresh turkey and I'm not going to freeze it." So, Irene cooked her turkey and made some gravy, and we made a cauliflower salad for the caretakers. Then we were one hour late getting to the hospital because the turkey took longer to cook than we expected, so everyone had already eaten. We have lots of delicious turkey left over. Hilary ate nothing. Tony didn't come because of his cold. What a bummer cold!

After the food was put away, we played Phase 10 with Ruth and Rick, the patient next to Hilary's room. It really did feel like Thanksgiving because we ate until we were uncomfortable, and then we played cards.

Yesterday, Hilary had her antifungal medicine so it was a quiet day. The mouth sores are a little better, but her throat is still really sore and her lower black lip looks awful. (She got a blood blister on her lower lip.) Rick is on day seven. He is walking many laps in the hall and looks very, very strong. Willie is just a little fatigued. Both of them still have hair and can eat almost anything. I'm glad everyone doesn't react like Hilary to their treatment. Michael is fighting nausea, so they haven't let him go yet. He is frustrated!

Love, Jan

Katie is now at the motel. Tabitha gets her transplant on Monday. Matt stays by himself most of the time. Dr. Simic told me yesterday, "What an amazing group of patients are on the floor right now." She doesn't feel like she has to go to work, because they are all so wonderful. She bought one of Rhonda's CDs. She has noticed what I see in most Christians—hope, peace, joy, love. That fruit of the Spirit is very apparent on this floor. I hope she recognizes the source of what makes us so wonderful.

Of course, Willie and Rhonda are so cute with everyone and with each other. They tease and smile all the time. There isn't doom and gloom, but excitement for healing, encouragement, and concern for everyone. There is laughter in the hall, greetings of love, and hugs. These people are truly amazing. We are a family who is just getting to meet one another. I wish I could introduce Dr. Simic to all of you, the rest of our family, where she would see more Spiritual fruits. I think you would "blow her socks off."

Love,
Jan

WATCHING AND WAITING

Hilary update, day 14
01 December 2003

Hilary's running a temperature. I thought they were going to give her Amphotericin (the antifungal) every day, but they changed it to Voriconazole every day. I'm glad they're changing to Voriconazole, because Hilary tolerates it a whole lot better than "shake and bake." They call Voriconazole "the big guns," but because Hilary had a previous condition of fungus, they're sure the infection specialists will approve. They took another chest x-ray, trying to find the reason for the temperature. Maybe her counts (white cells) are starting to come in.

They also started Ativan and Phenergan for nausea full-time. Hilary can ask for more if she feels the need, but because she vomited this morning and couldn't keep down her liver meds at 11:00 A.M., she took more nausea meds. Compazine to the rescue.

Hilary's mouth is better. The black scab on her lower lip keeps bleeding (so they gave her platelets), she is talking now, so one part of her throat is better, but the rest of her throat is still raw. She goes through a routine before anything enters her mouth: saline mouthwash, another saline mouthwash, special mouthwash with a numbing agent, more saline mouthwash, a push of the pain-medication button, a bite or sip of nourishment or liver medications in sherbet, and then another washing with saline mouthwash. I'm glad it is day 14. Waiting and watching, waiting and watching, waiting and watching. The end is coming.

Because her mouth is so much better, the nurses seem to think that some engraftment is taking place. I guess those white cells go right to work, die in the mouth and throat, and they don't show in the bloodstream until a million or so are present. Because her mouth is better, that is a sign improvement is around the corner.

It is now Tuesday morning and I'm at the apartment: Hilary slept yesterday away. After her second bout of nausea, Kris, her nurse brought in Compazine and it knocked Hilary out. When she awoke five hours later, her stomach hurt. I thought maybe a little yogurt would help. When Emily, the night nurse came on, she explained that the stomach and esophagus are sloughing off dead cells, just like the mouth did, and so maybe yogurt wasn't a good thing. Oh, being a stupid mom is just my cup of tea. I see my girl getting weaker, in spite of TPN (liquid food put through the PICC line). Her weakness is probably because of a temperature but I think in my sieve-like brain that nourishment could help. Then, my sweet Hilary eats just to please me and hurts just a little more. I'll find out when I get back to the hospital if it came back up and burned the raw throat in the process.

Emily understood my mom mentality. She had a very ill daughter at one time and almost did cartwheels after one bite of SpaghettiO's.

Waiting and watching...waiting and watching...waiting and watching. Guess what we are doing right now? Waiting and watching...waiting and watching. If she didn't have a temperature right now, the waiting and watching wouldn't be so bad.

I hope the temperature is because the immune system is going to work and causing a little heat in the process. How many meds can this hospital produce to correct the evil bacteria, virus, and fungus? Will they have a medicine for this temperature? We're waiting for the blood cultures to come back. The x-ray was clean. We're waiting for baby stem cells to save us. You know all this waiting business fits in perfectly with the attitude we are supposed to have during Advent. Waiting and watching, waiting and watching. Maybe if my sieve-like mind can remember this feeling, Advent will never be the same. A baby came to save us! Wow, what a thought. Baby stem cells...baby Jesus...both came to save us. A baby came to save us! Wow!

Got to go. Hilary just called and talked with Gabrielle. She did run a temperature throughout the night. Gabe didn't ask if the yogurt stayed down. Tony just called to say he's going to the hospital today. Finally! Yippee! Won't Hilary be surprised to see him? That should help the waiting and watching. It is a lot better waiting and watching at the hospital than watching and waiting from a distance. Talk to you later.

Love,
Jan

STILL WAITING

Hilary update, day 16
03 December 2003

Wednesday morning: Just a quick note...no counts yet. Everyone seems to think that some white cells are present, because Hilary's mouth is so much better. Her lower lip is normal again. Her throat is better. She is still running a temperature, but they are monitoring it very closely. If her temperature continues today, they'll probably do a CAT scan of her sinuses. Maybe the temperature is just sleepy stem cells going to work. Maybe tomorrow!

Love you,
Jan

WHITE CELLS

Hilary update, day 17
04 December 2003

We've got white cells! At 2:15 A.M., Hilary got a dandy bloody nose and when I went to tell the nurse about it, she handed me a copy of the midnight blood labs. Hilary's while cell count shows 0.2. Karen, the head night nurse, said, "Now don't start the white cell-count dance yet. It's not uncommon for the white cell count to show some activity and then disappear because they are working elsewhere."

I don't care; I'm doing the white cell-count dance. I've told everybody. I know a 0.2 white blood count (WBC) proves a functioning bone marrow is beginning. Progress is coming "little by little." The day is coming when the blood labs will no longer say A-negative blood type. It will declare Hilary has B-negative blood.

Hilary is sleeping a ton! I think her body is working really hard! Today she will have a CAT scan of her sinuses and her lungs because of her persistent fevers. The health team doesn't think they'll see anything, but want to make sure everything is still clear. Fevers are common for people during engraftment.

Michael got to go to the motel yesterday. I was excited for him, but wondered how he was doing. I was wishing I had a phone number to call just to check on him. It is amazing how we adopt each other. Then just a few minutes ago, here he comes to visit. Apparently, he got his

PICC line dressing wet in the shower and needed to come to clinic to be redressed, so he came over to check on Hilary. She, of course, was sleeping. Cindy, his mom, commented on how scary it was to do his IV. I remembered how anxious we all are to leave this secure, safe place, how the weight of responsibility seems to be extra intense. I compare it to the same excited nervousness of taking your one-day-old firstborn child away from the hospital. Big responsibility!

Please pray that they will find a donor for Michael. He received his own stem cells because he didn't have a donor. He has AML, just like Hilary and Matt. Hilary and Matt each had a transplant last year within a month of each other. Matt used his own stem cells and Hilary used Gabrielle's stem cells, which was like using her own. Both of them are here now receiving their second transplant using an unrelated donor.

I'm worried for Michael! Cindy told me today, after Michael went to visit Willie, that they are giving him only a 10 percent chance of not relapsing. I'm so glad Lizzie did a drive at Linfield a couple of weeks ago. Keep working at those donor drives. Especially encourage Hispanics, Asians, Native Americans, and African Americans to get involved. Michael has Hispanic and Italian background in his heritage.

While Michael and Cindy were here, Gail came to say hi while her Mike visited the clinic. Then Tom came over for a few minutes while Katie was in the clinic. These visitors of previous patients declare healing health. The ending is in sight.

Rick is doing so well that they are considering a possible release this coming weekend. Willie has some white cells showing, but he is battling those awful mouth sores. Matt is also battling mouth sores. Tabitha received her brother's stem cells Tuesday and looks absolutely beautiful.

Hilary and I just read day 17 in our book *The Purpose Driven Life*, and it talks about being members of a church body. It made me homesick for Eastern Oregon. Hilary mentions fairly often how she misses Bill's sermons. I miss all of you, but we are meeting distant Christian relatives while we are here. Father Jim from St. Elizabeth's is so good to come and see Hilary, always bringing communion with him. He has convinced me that I need to go to their Advent celebration this coming Friday, just to get away from the hospital. Father Jim has a big job ministering to this hospital. I saw him a couple nights ago (about 7:30 in the evening) walking across the sky bridge toward the VA hospital, looking very fatigued. He told me it had been a rough day and asked me to pray for a boy who was very much alone, even with family around him. Many, many hurting people he saw that day, and I saw their pain in his tired eyes.

Tabitha's church family has been here two or three times praying for all of us. They gave Hilary some anointed oil to rub on her body. I'm getting better about praying more openly because of these confident Christians surrounding me. My lessons never end in this journey with my wonderful, loving Jesus. It is fun meeting extended Christian family, visiting with wonderful nurses, being able to pray a little longer than just the car drive between Richland and Baker. I feel joy. Isn't that amazing? Maybe it's the confidence that I see God's promises in those cute little white cells. May you also find something to celebrate. Feel fruitful joy, smile.

Love,
Jan

WHITE CELL DANCE

Hilary update, day 18
05 December 2003

When Emily came on duty last night, she was excited about the 0.2 white cell count. She also said that she doesn't dance the white cell dance until the count is 0.3 and wondered if she should wake us when the midnight labs returned with the new results. Hilary and I both said that waking us wouldn't change the number, so we would see it in the morning. Well, of course, Hilary wakes often during the night and Emily

173

did the count dance at around 2:00. Then when I woke at 4:00, she had to do the dance again. Hilary's count was at 0.4.

This morning Karen taught me again how to figure the absolute neutrophil count (ANC). That count needs to be at 500 before anyone can leave the hospital and Hilary's ANC today is 220. Dr. Leis told the nurse to lessen the pain meds on the PCA so that Hilary could be off the PCA by tomorrow. He told Hilary to eat and drink often (she needs to take in two liters of fluid before they will let her depart), exercise often, breathe deeply often. It's time to get off the TPN. It's time to move on! The birth is over and now the work begins. Every new mom remembers that work of sleepless nights, and washing diapers and bedding and clothes and baby and…oh the joy of new life.

I promised Hilary I would only suggest fluid ideas and write down her count. She has to do this work and my constant reminding will only cause a fight. She's good at saying, "Maybe later," which means, "Back off, Mom." Boy is that hard for a control mom to do. How do I nudge/encourage an adult child to do the right thing without pushing the communication voice into a fight?

If things move along well, I think Hilary will be able to escape sometime next week. Won't that be wonderful? Now we need to start looking for signs of GVH. I asked Matt why he had used his own stem cells last year. I thought they probably couldn't find a donor for him. He told me he wanted to use his own stem cells because he didn't want to deal with GVH. Unfortunately, here he is anyway. From what I understand, the GVH should be over in a couple of years. It's just growing pains. I just pray that Hilary doesn't skin her knees too often while she learns to walk with her GVH.

Talk to you tomorrow.

Love,
Jan

LITTLE BY LITTLE

Hilary update, days +19 and 20
07 December 2003

I thought I should put the + before 19. That is the way it is written on the board by the nurses' desk. Patients who receive stem cells from an unrelated donor need to be fifteen minutes from the hospital for +100 days. Most people can leave the hospital around +20 days. Then they need to rent a motel room, or stay with friends and relatives until +100. I'm so glad that when Hilary leaves the hospital we have the apartment. Because yesterday's count was so wonderful, people from the clinic stopped me in the outside halls saying, "Wow! I saw the count. Wonderful!"

Since we've been through this before, everyone already knows Hilary's name and remembers her data. Today's white cell counts are still 0.4, but Hilary's absolute neutrophil count (ANC) was 120. That's down a few points. "That happens," as Hilary says. Yesterday, I told you that patients need a 500 ANC count to be released from the hospital. Oops, wrong. Bone marrow transplant patients need 500 ANC for two days before the team considers engraftment in place, and then they need 1000/1500 ANC for two days before a discharge is granted. A 0.4 white cell count is 400 white cells. To mathematically figure the ANC number, you add the percentage of neutrophils to the percentage of bands, and multiply that by the white cell count. Guess what I do every morning after the lab results arrive?

When Dr. Leis came in yesterday, I think he forgot that Hilary had a cord blood donor and the engraftments for cords are much slower than for adult stem cells. When the adult stem cells start engrafting, they seem to double each day. The Dornbecker doctor, who has used cord blood donors with children, told Hilary not to be surprised if her counts just "hang" for a while. They may even drop before growing again. That's OK, because Hilary is going to need some time to eat enough calories to remove the TPN and drink the daily enormous two liters of fluids. Besides, she is still on the PCA, which also has to be eliminated. They are giving less pain medication using the PCA, so everything is progressing. Another reason the PCA is still in place is because Hilary is having some strong stomach pains just below her ribs. She says it feels like heartburn. The nurses seem to think it is mucositis (like the mouth sores) in her stomach. That will take a few days to heal. So here is the intake report: our fighting warrior has improved her fluid intake from 2.6 oz. to over 15 oz. yesterday. If she doesn't swallow a bit more today, she won't match yesterday's amount. She has improved her calorie intake from zero to three bites of yogurt, two bites of potatoes, two bites of Tabitha's sister's wonderful soup, one bite of sausage, and almost half of an apple so far today. She walked on the treadmill for thirty minutes and stayed awake to watch a movie. I'm proud of her! Isn't it strange that only people who are trying to gain weight or lose weight check every bite that enters this marvelous body? What a battle it is either way!

Some of you have asked about the CAT scan. The CAT scan was clear. Praise God.

Ruth and Rick left today. They gave us a book called *Leaping* by Brian Doyle, and this author mentions that people write because writing is a form of contemplation but I write so I can clear my head. You are kind enough to not make fun of my rambles. Thank you.

This next week is finals. Elizabeth is finished on Tuesday and will probably be here on Thursday. Todd has his tough final on Tuesday and will be finished with everything by Thursday. Gabrielle and Tony's anatomy and physiology class final is Friday from 4:00 to 6:00. That's the class that seems to cause sleepless nights. Then we'll all be together "watching and waiting" for baby white cells.

Day 20

I didn't get this sent yesterday, so today's math problem revealed an ANC of 384. "Little by little" and "watch and wait" seem to be the lessons of this season. Willie's ANC is over 1000. He will probably get to go to their apartment tomorrow. Matt has 0.2 white cells today.

I met a new gentleman from Hermiston, who graduated from Baker High School in 1971. He moved into Rick's old room and will have a transplant in a few days. A lady who had a transplant five years ago came to give gifts to everyone on the floor. A payback of gifts she received five years ago. I wonder if Hilary will want to do something like that when she is finished with all of this.

Love you all bunches!

Talk to you later.

Love,

Jan

ANC 812

Hilary update, day +21
08 December 2003

The ANC today was 812. Isn't that great? She is working hard at the eating and drinking. If things keep improving, we might be at the apartment by the weekend.

Willie is going to their apartment today. Matt's counts are 0.7 Tabitha ate pizza for lunch. God is good!

Love,

Jan

ANC 1680

Hilary update, days +22 and +23
Wednesday, 10 December 2003

The ANC is 1680. Hilary is off the TPN and came off her last IV antibiotic. I'm thinking we might be able to go to the apartment by Friday. We'll see how much food and drink this girl can retain in the next couple of days. I stayed at the apartment to "clean" the bedroom today, preparing for a homecoming. Hilary's first question after Dr. Leis mentioned, "Maybe you'll be able to go home by the end of the week," was, "Is my bedroom clean?" I thought I'd get on the job, so Hilary would know we are ready for the big move.

Nothing else is happening for Hilary and me. Boring is wonderful! Everyone else seems extra busy. It is finals week for the students who live in our apartment complex.

The nurses are really hopping today. I don't know what is going on because of patient confidentiality, but I think the gentleman in the room at the end of the hall is really sick. We haven't met him, even though he has been here as long as Hilary. His day on the board is +76, but when I walk by his room, he is always lying with his back to the door. He looks like he is sleeping. When his caregiver is in the hall, she is on the cell phone.

Hilary and I spend our time reading and watching movies. We have our meals packed in to us. Theresa, the house cleaner, dumps our garbage and mops our floor. Doesn't that sound like a vacation?

Day +23

The ANC was 2823 today. Dr. Leis said maybe Hilary can leave this joint tomorrow. Wouldn't that be something! All of Hilary's blood counts are looking good, except platelets. They can watch those numbers at the clinic and give needed platelets when necessary. A couple of days ago, Hilary's platelets were 3 (a normal platelet count is above 140). Just a bit low, don't you think? On Monday, when her platelets were around 12, she got a bloody nose that lasted forty-five minutes. They ordered platelets from the Red Cross, but because the Red Cross was so low in platelets, it took six hours before a unit came. Tony called the Red Cross and gave an apheresis donation today. Todd plans to donate tomorrow. Tony had a letter from the Red Cross requesting a donation because they only had a one-day supply on hand. Maybe those of you who live in the Portland area might consider donating. Platelets don't live very long, so more platelet donations are needed more often.

Let me tell you about the Romanian youth group who came to visit Tabitha last Sunday. Tabitha invited everyone on the floor to come and join the prayer and worship time. Let me tell you about two interesting observations. First, the youth group consisted of at least fifteen people and they were mostly boys, with only three girls. I've noticed that our American youth groups are mostly girls. Second, the leader would explain what they were going to pray about, and then everyone started praying very loudly, all in Romanian. It was very fun! I'll write again when we are at the apartment!

Love to you all.

Jan

Chapter 11

APARTMENT HOME

Hilary update, day +25

12 December 03

It is 6:00 in the morning and we are at the apartment! We got home around 3:30 yesterday afternoon. Taking an inventory of our medical supplies was the first task at hand. I convinced the home health people to *not* send any more supplies until we understood what we already possessed. We still have boxes of medicine in our refrigerator from last year's fungal fight, which is worth about $1,000. They can't/won't take it back. I would even give it to them, but they think the plastic sealed containers have to be contaminated because it was out of their sight. What a waste! Government rules are sometimes stupid!

Then Hilary needed to take an inventory of prescription medicines before we ran to the pharmacy to fill all the new ones. After those tasks, our new immune system girl took a long shower, followed by a nap, after which she sat on the couch smiling while Elizabeth and Marissa challenged Gabrielle with anatomy and physiology questions. Gabrielle and Tony's big final is today. Gabe has had trouble focusing and needs an A on this final.

Today, Hilary needs to visit the clinic. They want to keep a close watch on the platelet count, not to mention all those other numbers found in the blood. We'll need to leave around 8:00 and plan on a "clinic" visit. Clinic visits can be one hour to six hours, depending upon the numbers in the lab report. A patient always plans for six hours. Patients learn to bring a lunch, books to read, letters to write, etc. When you plan on a six-hour visit and get to come home within two hours, a celebration erupts.

Hilary now has the battle of eating and drinking, which is similar to many other people in the U.S. I want her to write down her fluid and calorie intake, but I'm not sure she is going to agree. She didn't fill her "tool" box (the pill box given to her yesterday). She plans to keep all her prescription meds in a cute bowl, just like before. I wonder if this behavior shows a denial of illness or an attitude of health building.

All this thinking about food causes a person to ponder, "Give us this day our daily bread." Hope your battles are contained.

Prayerfully.

Love,

Jan

LOST PURSE

Hilary update, day +26
Saturday, 13 December 2003

"And days are like that. Even in Australia."[12] (From Judith Viorst *Alexander and the Terrible, Horrible, No-Good, Very Bad, Day.*) Yesterday was one of those days. As we were walking out the door to the clinic, Hilary asked, "Where is my purse?"

We did a quick search and decide it might still be in the trunk of the car. When we got to the clinic, we did a search of the trunk...no purse. As Hilary waited for the lab report, I took the car for an inside vacuuming. No purse. Then I walked to 5C to ask if we'd left it in the room. Nope, we didn't. Next stop was the security, which houses the lost-and-found department for OHSU campus. No purse. So then we called the apartment to have Gabrielle and Tony take a break from studying to look for the purse. Couldn't find it. I went back and looked in the trunk one more time. Then I remembered putting a sack of Hilary's clean clothes in her closet, but I hadn't unloaded it. Called the apartment again and asked them to check that sack. Yes, it was there!

After clinic, Hilary was extra weak and a bit white around the eyeballs, so we walked arm in arm back to the car. When we got to the car, it wouldn't start. I thought it might be a dead battery, so we called the apartment again to let them know we were now sitting in the parking lot. Elizabeth came to the rescue, because Gabrielle and Tony needed to leave for their final test in anatomy and physiology.

Elizabeth rolled into the parking lot and bumped a truck, which broke the cover on her turn-signal light. No damage was caused to the truck. The lights still worked on Elizabeth's car, so home we went. We made it home fine, then I cut my finger while cooking supper. Yes, "some days are like that."

The day ended with a Christmas concert at George Fox College. Elizabeth, Gabrielle, and I went while Tony and Hilary stayed at the apartment. The concert, by the way, was absolutely awesome!

I'm surprised that during the valleys and mountains of this day, I didn't feel distraught. Is that a sign of maturity or a result of all your prayers? Either way, I know Jesus is the cause of leveling emotions... hope your mountains and valleys are leveled.

Love,

Jan

Steroids

Hilary update, day +35
Monday, 22 December 2003

Hilary is strengthening "little by little." Last Friday's clinic lasted from 8:30 until 5:00. Then she walked to the car without needing Mom for a crutch. This event was a wonderful marker of growth for this mom, who doesn't always notice the "little by little" changes. Hilary's clinic schedule has been Tuesdays, Fridays, and Sundays. The clinic blood tests are part of Hilary's immune system. The blood cultures look for any evil germs. The steroids suppress the immune system (GVH control) and the body might not notice those evil germs, so the blood tests look for them. Hilary receives a magnesium replacement infusion on her clinic dates because the steroids wash magnesium from the body. Hilary takes a sleeping pill every night, because the steroids make her agitated and cause sleepless nights.

As you can see, these steroids are very important, but they do cause some dandy side effects. The clinic's blood labs check the levels (counts) for everything: white cells, red cells, platelets, liver enzymes, kidney function, potassium, magnesium, plus a bunch of other stuff including the levels of steroids. We were so excited that Hilary could lower her dose of steroids last Friday.

As for our normal days (non-clinic days), we are busy doing normal activities: cooking, cleaning, and preparing for Christmas. I've been pondering when to return to work. Tony is shopping for a dependable car. Aunt Peggy and Grandpa came to visit for a few days. Had an opportunity to meet Earl, Christy's baby—another miracle in which God has used medicine to provide healing. Watching each of us take turns holding him, smiling in awe at the wonderment of his charm and innocence, caused me to ponder how Mary held and adored baby Jesus. If I can remember that feeling of holding Earl, that feeling of wonderment and adoration, maybe I'll take time to adore Jesus more this Christmas.

Life is good…boring is good…friends and family are wonderful…parking is great for weekend clinics…had an hour to read stuff from www.gospel.com, a wonderful site…yoga is fun…so much to be thankful for…so much to be joyful about…our lives are blessed indeed. Thank you for being part of our blessed life. Praying you'll have time to adore Jesus, our daily bread, and notice His wonderful blessings in being normal.

Love you all bunches! Consider this e-mail our Christmas carol singing and imagine you are eating some of our Christmas cinnamon bread.

Love you,

Jan

FROZEN PIPES

Hilary update, day 55
10 January 2004

Day 55, but who's counting? It's hard to believe Hilary is over the halfway mark to the honored 100 days! Her blood counts are continuing to climb or are staying normal. Two of her liver counts (the SGOT and SGPT) are high, but because the total bilirubin is in the normal range, the team doesn't think the GVH is attacking the liver. They took away the antifungal medicine and lowered the GVH medicines to see if the liver counts will drop. They have also started Hilary on marijuana (a pill form) to try to increase her appetite. She is holding around 95 pounds, and when the scale dropped three pounds, concern for weight gain became immediate. Other than that, she is doing "boring" activities! Isn't that wonderful?

I went home to Richland last Saturday. Elizabeth and I came through The Gorge on Friday, where the roads were absolutely awful around Hood River. It took an hour to travel ten miles. It was nice to get to

Boardman, where the roads were better and traffic less congested. I stayed in La Grande on Friday night, and then I visited with my substitute about school before driving on into Richland Saturday afternoon. Monday morning, my class was surprised at having me back, but I didn't hear, "Oh, Mrs. Bonn, it's so nice for you to be back...welcome home....we missed you...etc." (The other teachers said those words, but my class didn't.) My class also didn't indicate, "Yuk, Mrs. Bonn is back," which would have broken my heart. Maybe they are just so used to my being gone, and they enjoy my substitute so much, that life is "boring."

About 8:30 Monday evening, we started losing water pressure at home. Because Tony is still in Portland, I knew it was up to me to find the frozen pipe and get it fixed. Earlier, Tony said it would probably be a good idea to put a second lightbulb in the pump house, in case the first bulb burned out. That was the first place to look. I called Dad to make sure he wasn't going to bed yet, just in case I would need help beyond the pump house. He said to take an electric heater to the pump house. Thus, I gathered my supplies of a large, 24-inch flashlight, two lightbulbs, and a small electric heater. I dressed with my big, heavy snow boots, a stocking hat, scarf, gloves, and work coat. Then I picked up the supplies, which I didn't put into a sack because I could hold them all in my arms.

When I got outside, the moon was so bright I didn't need the flashlight but decided to pack it anyway, just in case I needed it at the pump house. I arrived at the fence gate, and it was frozen shut. I kicked at it, but heard a slight crack. Since I wasn't sure if it was the wood breaking or the ice breaking, I decided to climb the fence rather than create the need to mend the gate. Now my dilemma of getting over the fence with my arms full of supplies and my boots slippery from snow became a joke. I managed a successful clamber, with a spell sitting on the top rail, knowing I had the other side to go down. I was glad that Jazz, my dog, didn't laugh at me but just wagged her tail in encouragement.

When I got to the pump house, I needed to empty my arms so I could open the door. Sure enough, the lightbulb was burned out and I exchanged it for a new one, and then put the second bulb in place for the backup. With my winter garb on, the pump house seemed warm, so I didn't leave the electric heater. Consequently, with the exception of one lightbulb, I began my descent to the house with my arms full of the same load I started with. The fence was easier to climb coming back and when I arrived back in my yard, I stopped to enjoy winter—the brilliant dark sky with the full moon's light reflecting off the smooth snow, the crispness of frosted air while my body was stuffed in a bundle of cloth, the noiseless space underneath speechless trees. My thoughts of laughter while sledding with Tony on Harris' Hill in Halfway strolled through my memory—wonderful winter, which I would have missed except for a burned out lightbulb and freezing pipes.

Love,

Jan

WINTER ROADS

Hilary update

25 January 2004

Hilary is blessed! Her liver enzymes are dropping. After removal of the marijuana, which the team used to stimulate appetite, the enzymes came creeping downward. Her magnesium level is holding better. Now she visits the clinic twice a week instead of three times. That is a small taste of freedom. Everything is fabulous. The only concern at this moment is her weight. She is 89 pounds. She is trying to eat and drink a ton, and no weight is gained. Tony is gaining weight trying to help Hilary gain weight. Hilary is active, so this skinny body isn't making her extra tired. She feels good. It would be marvelous, possibly necessary, to have some weight increase in case the ugly GVH shows up. She might need to have a weight advantage for the fight.

Love, Jan

My roads have been very nice and dry with a few patches of ice. Then on Friday morning, Mr. Winter decided to return from vacation and add to the snow on the hills. He blew snow in whips of fog like fuzz across the road. The herd of elk that were behind the barn this last week were milling in the road, trying to decide which side looked greener (only white was to be viewed).

Then, Friday evening, the road had packed snow with lots of deer munching on the brush along the side. Elizabeth told me that EOSC (Eastern Oregon State College) closed at 2:00 on Friday because of freezing rain. I'm glad we got snow. By today I have a sore back from shoveling a foot of snow from my front walk and around my car.

I wish I had some kids around to make a snow fort or create a sled run on the hill. Dad plowed my driveway after church. I'm glad, because when I drove back into my shoveled car spot, I filled my headlights with snow while dragging the bottom of my car. If this snow froze solid, I might break something just trying to get to work. I hope winter decides to vacation again this week, so I can drive to Portland for the weekend. I want to cook in the Portland kitchen.

I hope this e-mails find you all eating well and enjoying Mr. Winter.

Love,
Jan

STONES

Hilary update, day 89
Saturday, 14 February 2004

Only eleven more days until the milestone day 100. Since things are going so wonderfully well, this will be the next-to-last Hilary update. What a long journey! What intense lessons! Thank you for sharing it with us by praying, and then praying some more.

188

Thank you again for all the support with your cards, phone calls, smiles, and hugs. I'm glad we're getting close to this milestone, but I realize that it is just that—another stone. Hilary's life will probably continue to include many doctor appointments, blood tests, CAT scans, etc., but that will be just a part of her path. We each have stones in our paths. Some stones we have to pack and some stones we have to climb over. The stones just look different. At least, I think that Hilary's stones will be smaller now and easier to climb over. The only stone she needs to pack is the problem of eating. At least she is gaining ounces each weigh-in day.

She is looking forward to eating a lettuce salad because her 100-day immune system could handle any hidden germs found in fresh greens. She is looking forward to starting school. She bought some expensive shampoo to wash her fuzzy head. She has pink in her cheeks, a bounce in her step and a smile on her face. She is beautiful! We are so wonderfully blessed!

We don't have results of the bone marrow biopsy yet, but Hilary thinks her donor is a girl. They needed to take more marrow than usual to check the chromosomes. (If the donor was a boy, it would be easy to see which cells were donor cells and which cells were still Hilary's cells.) We're planning to visit Germany sometime in the future, in hopes to meet this little girl. Won't that be fun! Hilary and Gabrielle are planning a huge twenty-first birthday party in November. I'll send you all an invitation. It will be another milestone.

As I've thought about this experience, I've decided that health is a gift. We think we have control of our health. We think the doctors are miracle-makers, but health is a gift from God. We truly have no control. Hilary's last neighbor at the hospital is no longer walking with us. I went to see him on Super Bowl Sunday and shook his hand while I told him I was praying for him. He seemed so confident that what the doctors were doing next to fight his fungus infection was going to work. Then I got an e-mail on Wednesday of that week telling me he was gone. I cried. I cried tears of sadness that his wife and nine-year-old daughter

Love, Jan

would not have him around for advice. I cried tears for his students, who will miss his encouragement. I related to his life. He was a teacher who graduated from Baker High School. He lived and worked in Eastern Oregon. I met his family and knew some of his friends. I cried tears of guilt because Hilary is still with us and we did nothing to deserve this. Hilary is no better than any other person who has leukemia. Why is she doing so well? It is a gift. I remember her saying when she was fighting the fungus infection, "Mom, everything will be all right. Don't worry. All worry does is ruin today. If I live, I'm all right. If I die, I'm all right. Everything will be all right."

I just know I would be so lonesome without her around. I'm so glad God chose the first, living "all right" and not the second, heaven "all right." Would I be angry with God if he had chosen to give Hilary the gift of health in heaven? I don't know. I'm glad that stone wasn't for me to climb. I'm glad the promise is this living picture of health. Praise to Jesus, the rock of salvation, who helps us climb over the large stones in our path.

May your life be full of small stones.

Love,

Jan

DAY 100

Hilary update, day 100
Sunday, 29 February 2004

This is it, my last Hilary update. Isn't that wonderful that Hilary is becoming boring? We have certainly felt carried by your prayers. We have met some wonderful people who became our teachers, our supporters, our motivators. Some of those people are you. Mel Gibson said during an interview about his movie *The Passion*, "Pain is a precursor to change."[13] We have changed. I have changed. And your prayers have been part of that change. Thank you!

190

Today I read Mark's story about Jesus healing a blind man. After such a dramatic change, "Jesus sent him home with the order, 'Don't go back into the village'" (Mark 8:26). I don't want to go back to my worried, fearful life. I want to continue to know Jesus as I know him now. I pray I will continue to grow without needing the pain of Hilary's suffering to prompt my changing.

As for the wonderful 100th day! Hilary celebrated with a lettuce salad at Red Robin. Irene and Tony were with her. Then she got an upset stomach. Isn't that typical of celebrations using food? Her real celebration came the weekend before, when the clinic allowed her to leave that tether of twenty minutes from the hospital to go to La Grande to watch Pine Eagle girls play basketball. I wish she could have watched last night's stressful, exciting, two-overtimes, two-point winning game against Umatilla, qualifying the team to go to state. I hope the girls win again on Wednesday so Hilary can go and watch them on Friday. Hilary still cannot drive, so she is limited to the chauffeuring of other people and their schedules. I debated traveling to Portland to celebrate Hilary's 100th day with her, but decided that celebrations should happen every day, not just on special days. Do I need to go to Portland on that particular day, when I celebrate every trip to Portland?

I am going down for the appointment with Dr. Fleming in March. I think he'll tell us that Hilary is doing wonderfully—beyond medical expectations—but, she'll need to do two more chemo treatments to her brain, watch for cataracts in her eyes, keep looking out for GVH problems, etc. If he has a message that puts me into a tailspin, even though I said this was my last e-mail, you'd better believe I'll be crying for more supportive prayerful help. How can I ever convince all of you that prayers are tangible hands supporting those of us who are stumbling in the dark?

Last Thursday, Gabrielle took Hilary to visit East West School of Massage. Hilary is applying for scholarships in order to start school in October. Because her energy level is still really low, she cannot work if she goes to school full-time, which she will need to do in order to receive any of those scholarships. I know that everything will work out. By October, she will have the energy to fulfill her dreams.

Allow me to leave you with some vocal snapshots that have run through my head periodically since Hilary started this journey:

Medical personnel in Alaska: "It looks like a wicked virus of some sort."

Overhearing the nurse on the Med/Surg. floor in Alaska talking to the pulmonary specialist: "I can't have a person coding on me up here. I don't have enough staff to take care of a person with a 104 temperature and a continuing oxygen level of 82 percent!"

ICU staff in Alaska: "Sorry ma'am, but you need to stay out there until we have her in place. You can watch from here."

Tony on the phone: "I'll be there tonight!"

While I sat in Alaska beside Hilary's ICU bed, watching Hilary sleep at 4:00 in the morning, an angel came and stood at the foot of Hilary's bed. I was convinced that the angel was there to take Hilary to heaven. In fear I asked, "Why are you here?" The angel's answer: "I'm here to watch the monitor with you." I sighed. After a long pause, the angel said, "She will be all right."

Tony's response: "What does 'all right' mean? She would be all right if she was in heaven."

Dr. Stewart: "We got the results of the bone marrow biopsy, and this isn't a virus but leukemia."

Dr. Janis, infection specialist: "At least we now know what we are fighting."

Elizabeth: "It's really hard when people give you mini-heart attacks by saying, 'You need to call your Aunt Kathy as soon as you can.'"

Aunt Mary at OHSU, while Hilary was gagging on the intubation tube: "Hilary, you're floating on a cloud. It's so comfortable. It's warm and cozy. The sun is shining. You can breathe easily. You're floating and comfortable." (Hilary was so good at this visualization that the gagging stopped. I was so glad Mary was there!)

Mark L. on 5C: "Now is the time to plant your roots deep into whatever faith you have. Don't go searching for anything new; just plant deep."

Sandra S., telling us to read Psalm 91:14–16 (TEV), where God says, "I will save those who love me and will protect those who acknowledge me as Lord. When they call to me, I will answer them; when they are in trouble, I will be with them. I will rescue them and honor them. I will reward them with long life; I will save them." (I read these words daily for two months and then tonight's responsorial psalm was this reading...wonderful words!)

The Upper Room devotional based on Mark 6:45–52 where Jesus was going to pass them by, but they saw him walking on the water... they were all terrified...then he got into the boat with them and the wind died down.

Isaiah 53:5(TEV): "But because of our sins he was wounded, beaten because of the evil we did. We are healed by the punishment he suffered, made whole by the blows he received."

Lord's Prayer: "Give us this day our daily bread."

Mark L.: "I'm sorry you have to go through this valley, but I'm also excited because you will get a closeness to our Lord that is irreplaceable."

The melody of Marty Haugen's song based on Psalm 23 embedding itself into a prayer as I repeat the refrain over and over.

Hilary's 100th day was on Ash Wednesday. Isn't that something! Now when the priest rubs ashes on my head and says, "Remember that thou art dust, and to dust thou shalt return," I will be thanking God for allowing Hilary's "all right" to mean 100 days past transplant. I don't know how to end...except to just stop typing...thanks for all your prayers.

Love,

Jan

Love, Jan

TIME TO CELEBRATE

Hilary update
Monday, 25 October 2004

Hilary asked me to send the following message to all in the address book:

You are invited to a birthday party! A year ago Gabrielle and I were spending our second consecutive birthday in the hospital. A couple of doctors said that for our twenty-first they would come visit us *out* of the hospital. Well, the time has come and we're going to hold them to it. On Friday, November 19th, 2004, Gabrielle and I are going to celebrate our twenty-first birthday! And *you* are invited!

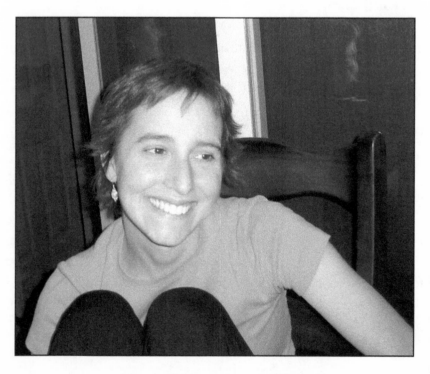

Hilary and Gabrielle's 21st Birthday.

Chapter 12

January 21

Hilary update
21 January 2005

Well, I wish this update was good news. Hilary went into the hospital last night. She is currently in ICU with double pneumonia. She has been intubated, so a machine is breathing for her. As of now I'm being told it is bacterial pneumonia, which is much better than viral. More tests are being done all the time. She is sedated and sleeping.

Thank you in advance for your prayers, not only for Hilary and her quick healing but for Jan, Tony, Irene, Elizabeth, and Gabe. This family is remarkable and, as always, have rallied around our sweet Hilary. She will never be alone.

Aunt Peggy

Love, Jan

POSITIVE NUMBERS

Hilary update
26 January 2005

Baby steps...Hilary is taking very small baby steps, but at least her baby steps are going in the right direction. As of last night when I left, her peep was at 8 instead of 10 (that is the positive air flow to keep her alveoli open in order to help oxygen pass through), her oxygen was at 50 percent, which was up 5 percent from the night before; her oxygen saturation (sats) were staying above 90; respiration was in the 20s; heart rate was around 80; and blood pressure was above 60. Oh, I forgot—they took her off the blood pressure medication because she was keeping her own blood pressure up.

One of the tests came back positive for respiratory syncytial virus (RSV). So the doctors were right—this problem did not return with Irene's trip to Brazil, but came from right here in Portland. Because it is a virus, we are basically keeping Hilary comfortable and supported until her antibodies kick in. They are supporting an inflamed lung, waiting for the miracle of healing that God has placed in each of us already. RSV is very contagious and causes mild respiratory infections such as colds and coughs in adults, but in young children it can produce severe pulmonary diseases including bronchitis and pneumonia. More than half of all infants are exposed to RSV by their first birthday and many have few or no symptoms; however, some infants with RSV become very ill. RSV is the most common cause of bronchitis and pneumonia among infants and children under the age of one. Children with severe disease may require oxygen therapy and sometimes mechanical ventilation. (Can you tell those are words from some papers the nurse gave us?) Because Hilary's immune system is around the age of one, and a bit suppressed because of steroids, here we are.

We were moved to the seventh floor ICU on Monday night, and that evening of dropping blood sugars, dropping heart rate, dropping oxygen,

196

and dropping blood pressure was a teeth-chattering, knee-shaking experience. I couldn't believe how my body reacted. But when the nurse went (in a hurry) to get the respiratory therapist (RT), I gently grabbed Hilary's hand and asked her to not let her body fall down. Of course, the nurse had given Hilary a shot of dextrose just before she left for the RT, and Tony said that diabetic people in shock will become normal within minutes of some sugar intake. I'm sure the sugar and my hand touched Hilary at the same time, but regardless of the reason, Hilary's numbers returned. I like the nurses in ICU, but for the most part I'm very impressed with all the nursing care Hilary has received.

As for my emotions about the medical doctors, I got a lesson from our wonderful teacher Jesus/God. During my devotional time on Monday, I read about the women who went to the tomb early in the morning on the third day. After seeing the angels and no Jesus, they returned to the apostles to tell them what the angels said:

"Why are you looking among the dead for one who is alive? He is not here; he has been raised. Remember what he said to you while he was in Galilee: 'The Son of Man must be handed over to sinners, be crucified, and three days later rise to life.'"

—Luke 24:5–7

But the apostles thought that what the women said was nonsense, and they did not believe them.

—Luke 24:11

So, those poor women were dismissed because they were women. Just like we have been dismissed because we are just family. My lesson was wondering how those women reacted to the dismissal. Were they angry, like Tony and I? Did they complain to their friends? Or were they so excited about hearing the message of resurrection and so focused on their love for Jesus that the apostles' dismissal was unimportant? What really mattered was the truth of the event. So, what is the truth of this matter of Hilary's health, not my emotions? Where should my focus be?

Love, Jan

Then, after about four hours of reading and pondering these words from Luke, one main doctor who truly dismissed me earlier in the morning, came and apologized for his curtness. It was good to have already forgiven him because of my morning's lesson and not have to digest the apology at that time.

Oh, the lessons we learn while sitting in a hospital.

Please pray for Mark Lawer and family. Mark was admitted into the ICU the same time as Hilary was, and they took him home to die in his own home. He had his transplant during Hilary's first transplant, e-mailed her often, came to encourage her during the brain chloroma, and was an inspiration of faith. Mark taught me many truths about God. He told us to plant our roots deep. He gave Hilary a Bible, because on our first trip to OHSU we didn't have one with us. He explained that we would meet Jesus during the valleys (Psalm 23) in a way that no other place can reveal His love. He advised us about medical terms, and he always called Hilary "the Beloved of God." He and Teri prayed for her daily.

We sat with Teri, Mark's wife, while she questioned the reason God has for allowing this turn of events. How could Jesus be glorified in Mark's death? Mark isn't dying of leukemia; he is dying from GVHD and a sick world that carries virus, bacteria, and fungi. Teri just kept shaking her head about the coincidence that we started together on 5C, and we're in ICU together at this time. She said, "Hilary can get well now. She brought you here when I needed your support." Of course, we have not mentioned Mark or Teri while in Hilary's room, and Teri didn't ever come in to visit Hilary. Hilary seems to react to tension in a negative manner (oxygen level lowers) and so she only gets to hear how much she is loved by all of us. Even though she is asleep, she still reacts.

A cousin sent me words from Romans 8 about how the Spirit prays for us when we cannot speak words. *Amen.* Because my prayer words are repetitive..."Heal Hilary." Thank you for carrying us with your prayers.

Love,
Jan

Peggy's Note

Hilary update
28 January 2005, 11:54 A.M.

Hi, everyone. Thank you for your continued prayers. *Keep them coming.*

Jan can't get to a computer, so this update is from me, Aunt Peggy.

They changed the sedative on Hilary last night. It didn't work as well so she was agitated with the tube down her throat. The good news is she regained some consciousness. Jan was able to tell Hilary what was going on and how much we all love her. She nodded in understanding.

This morning she is back on the high dose of the other sedative. Other good news is her x-rays are showing improvement. Also, the latest test checking for a return of the leukemia came back negative. They have done a bone marrow test for additional confirmation but we won't have the results of that for about five days.

Thank you again for your prayers.

Aunt Peg

Hilary in Heaven

Hilary update
Friday, 28 January 2005

Friday, January 28, 2005. 8:30 P.M. Hilary passed away.

Peggy

Love, Jan

JANUARY 29

January 29, 2005

Hilary died Friday evening, January 28, at the OHSU ICU medical floor. Her leukemia returned just as it had started, as a pretended lung infection. Alaska couldn't find any problem two-and-a-half years ago in her blood, and only did a bone marrow test to rule out leukemia as a reason for this girl being so horribly sick. Then, OHSU couldn't understand why the antibiotics were not helping the awful pneumonia this girl exhibited. They did a bone marrow test to rule out leukemia as the reason for her pneumonia. A hundred years ago, or probably even fifty years ago, the coroner would have written on Hilary's death certificate: "Cause of death, pneumonia." We were told about the bone marrow results around 3:00, and Hilary's life support was removed around 6:00 P.M. She was asleep when the tubes were removed, and left us while sleeping around 8:30 P.M.

Throughout the week, I kept mixing the stories of the Roman officer asking for help for his servant and the Jewish official asking for help for his daughter. Jesus healed them both. I was thinking about our Catholic response at communion when we say, "I'm not worthy to receive you, but only say the word and we shall be healed." I wondered why Jesus wasn't saying "the word." He only had to say the word.

I remember Hilary not ever saying, "Why me?" about this leukemia. In fact, I think she told me once, "Why not me? Why should I be treated special?" My answer now would be, "Because you, sweetie, are extra special and deserve every reason to be treated special from the master healer, Jesus."

Well, I understand that every parent says the same thing. Judy said those words to me when Ryan was dying. Did Jesus treat Hilary in a special way? Well, I suppose he did. She never complained about pain. She didn't seem afraid of death or disease. She always had a calmness about her, and Luke 1:78 and 79 (TEV) says:

200

"Our God is merciful and tender. He will cause the bright dawn of salvation to rise on us and to shine from heaven on all those who live in the dark shadow of death, to guide our steps into the path of peace."

Hilary seemed to be at peace. That was the special way Jesus helped Hilary. She was excited about school, and most of the last week she slept through her pain. I have wondered about Lazarus, whom Jesus called from the grave after Lazarus had been in there three days. I had even hoped Jesus would surprise all of us and do another Lazarus miracle.

But in a way, Jesus gave us two and a half years of a Lazarus story. I know Lazarus isn't alive today, so after a period of time, he also died. I agree with my sister, Peggy, when she said, "I am so thankful for these last two and a half years. Hilary went through a miserable experience giving all of us time to learn, enjoy her company, and get ready to say good-bye."

Hilary's memorial is set for 6:00 P.M. on Thursday at the Richland Grade School. Everyone tells us that the Methodist Church just won't be large enough to hold everyone who wants to come. I know Hilary would want people to be comfortable, but I really wanted a homier, relaxed room—not a gym. But, with Lizzie's help, I'm sure this gym will be beautiful.

People have offered their bedrooms for those of you who have to travel a distance. Just let us know if you need a bed. We'll find you one. We're having a potluck in the cafeteria of the school after the memorial, just so we have a chance to visit and tell stories. My family heals their hearts by telling stories. These long-winded e-mails you've received for the last two years have been a healing for me. Thank you for listening to my e-mail stories. You've been healing my heart for a long time.

I'm attaching Nancy's note about the benevolence fund, for those of you who are interested. I love you all very much.

Jan

Love, Jan

Benevolence Fund/Richland Methodist Church

Jan has asked if I would try to let you know what the benevolence fund is all about.

When everyone was wondering how they could help Hilary and family a couple of years ago, there was a question of how to make a donation that could be tax-free and yet meet the needs that there could be for Hilary and family.

The Richland Methodist Church said that they would become the caretakers of a benevolence fund so donations are tax deductible. The benevolence fund is completely independent from the Methodist Church budget and 100 percent of the funds are used for those who are in need and ask for help. A board of directors makes the decisions about who receives the money and how much. All information is confidential. Request for funding can be addressed to:

Richland Methodist Church
P.O. Box 378
Richland, OR 97870

Make donations to this fund at the same address. Just make the check to:

Benevolence Fund/Richland Methodist Church.

Although this fund was set up with the money given in Hilary's name, Hilary felt very strongly that she wanted that money to be there for those in our communities who had a need. Money has been donated to the fund that has not been in Hilary's name, and so the fund continues to grow. The benevolence fund is there for people in need or to those who just need a boost with expenses that aren't covered by other means.

I know that Hilary was always excited when she heard that money had been given to someone who had a need. That was part of the beautiful spirit that made Hilary the special person she was. That spirit will live on through this fund and makes this a special fund.

If you have questions, feel free to call me at 541-893-6536, and I will try to answer your questions.

Nancy

Author's Notes

WHY AM I now compiling these e-mail messages into a book? Different people who were receiving these e-mails commented about combining them into a book. At first I was shockingly pleased that anyone would think a C-average English student could possibly be a writer. Then as more people made the same request, I started imagining the marvelous possibility. I envisioned how God could use Hilary's story to increase faith in his amazing ways. It was vanity.

When Hilary's story didn't end with the healing everyone wanted or what I expected, I wondered how God could be glorified with this kind of finish. How could other people's faith increase when my faith was shaken to its core? My cousin Debbie insisted that the story was still important for people who were experiencing a stem cell transplant. Yet I wondered if the end of this story would discourage anyone in the transplant process. People like winning! Hilary lost her fight with leukemia. But did she really lose life?

When I discussed the book idea with my sister Peggy, she mentioned that the book was really about me. Everyone has disappointments and life stresses. People want to read about trust in God. I worried that Hilary's story would not increase trust.

Love, Jan

Why am I now compiling these e-mail messages into a book? To increase funds for the Hilary Benefit account, to encourage hope and faith in the resurrected Jesus, to give an account of Hilary's stem cell transplant process for anyone who also needs to amble along that path, and I suppose a bit of vanity is also involved. My hope is Paul's words in Colossians 1:2:

"I do this in order that they may be filled with courage and may be drawn together in love and so have the full wealth of assurance which true understanding brings. In this way they will know God's secret, which is Christ himself."

This is my prayer, that you, the reader, may come closer to God's secret, which is Christ himself.

Epilogue

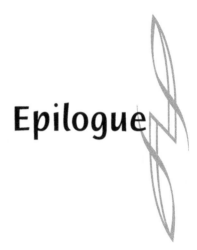

TONY AND GABRIELLE graduated as registered nurses in 2007. Even though Tony attended Treasure Valley Community College and Gabrielle attended Umpqua Community College, these colleges allowed Tony to stand with Gabrielle on the Umpqua stage in Roseburg, Oregon, so they could award each other their nursing pins in the pinning ceremony.

One year later, Gabrielle and Todd were married at Todd's family ranch with Bill Shields as the pastor. It was a glorious day. Gabrielle gave each of us lockets with small pictures of Hilary to wear. The surprise locket was tied into our corsages and boutonnière and caused the only tears Tony and I shared that day. Gabrielle currently works for a local hospital in Roseburg, Oregon.

In 2005, Elizabeth graduated from OHSU's nursing program hosted on La Grande's Eastern Oregon University campus. She had two nursing aunts travel to watch her pinning ceremony, along with Gabrielle, Tony, Grandpa, and me. At this time she is working in the IV therapy department in a hospital close to West Linn, Oregon. She has the opportunity to install PICC lines, those wonderful tubes that prevent much needle poking.

Irene married this last February in Hawaii. It was a lovely vacation while we watched a beautiful wedding on the beach at 7:00 in the morning. We all wore the Hilary lockets while the pastor started the wedding by talking about a great cloud of witnesses from heaven joining all of us during the blessed time of marriage. Irene presently works as a personal chef and yoga instructor. This unbiased mom thinks that Irene is unusually talented and people are fortunate when they are able to work with her.

Tony began working as a medical/surgical nurse in Baker City. He works night shift, which he enjoys. He continues to fix anything that breaks, helps with canning and cooking, and desires to protect all his girls. I am blessed to have such a wonderful man in my life.

I fill my life with music, movies, and muse while I read books, meander along walks, visit with friends, drive along the Powder River Canyon, and vacation with family. I continue my efforts to broaden children's minds in my classroom in Baker City. My life is abundant and blessed.

Jan Bonn

Richland, Oregon

January 2010

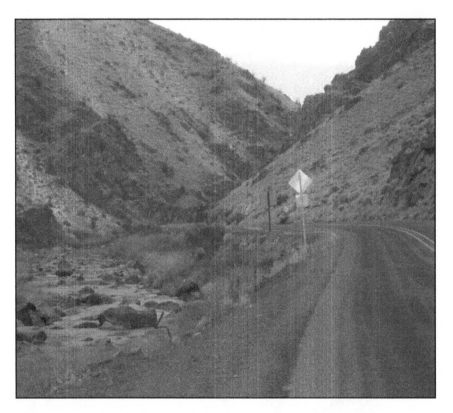

The Powder River road, a 40 mile distance, between Richland and Baker City.

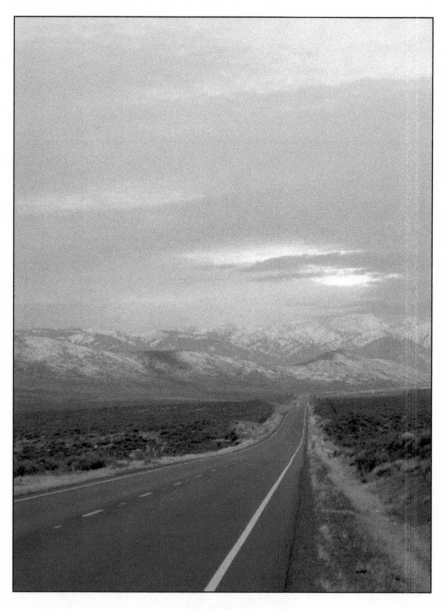

The Elkhorn Mountains hover over Baker City. They are a magnificent view for any traveler who maneuvers the Powder River road and a reminder of Psalms 121. "I look to the mountains, where will my help come from? My help will come from the Lord, who made heaven and earth." Psalms 121: 1&2

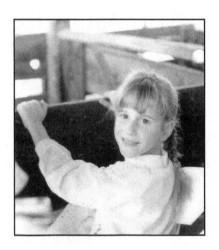

The Bonn Girls earned money for college raising 4-H lambs.
In this photo, Hilary is eight years old, standing on her lamb's pen gate
at the Halfway Fair.

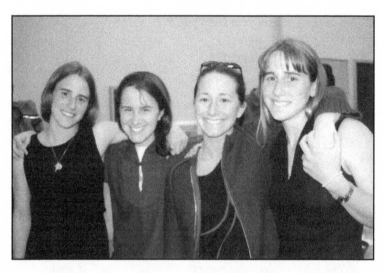

The Bonn Girls taken by Jennifer Godwin at a high school music/art event in 2001.

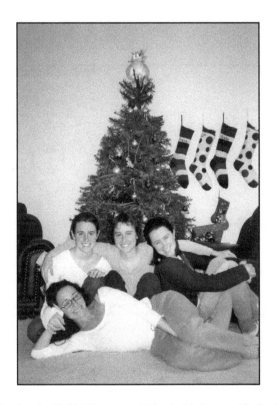

The Bonn Girls taken by Todd. These were Hilary's Christmas gifts for family in 2004.

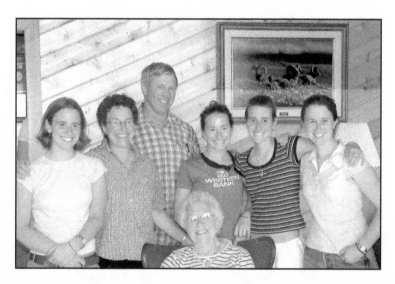

Anthony Bonn family taken with Grandma Irene at a Bonn family reunion, during the summer of 2003.

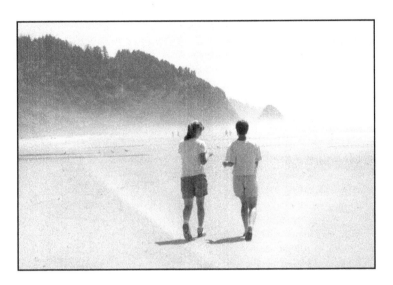

This is one of Jan's favorite pictures during one of the family's annual trips to the Oregon beach. Elizabeth took this picture of Hilary and Gabrielle in 2000.

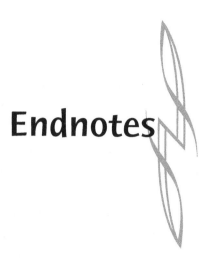

Endnotes

1. There are three main types of stem cell transplantation: *syngeneic, allogeneic,* and *autologous.* Syngeneic transplant is when the donor and recipient are identical twins. Since the genetic makeup is the same, this transplant would not be rejected or attacked by the donor's immune system. Allogeneic transplant is a transplant between two individuals with a tissue type very closely matched. Usually a sibling fits this matching because of the genetic composition of having the same parents. Compatibility is assessed by laboratory tests. If an unrelated donor is needed, one is usually found from the large pool of volunteers registered with the stem cell donor list. When an allogeneic transplant is used, there is the potential for immune rejection of the donated stem cells by the recipient, called *host versus graft.* Autologous transplant is really a therapy, a technique of obtaining stem cells from and returning stem cells to the same individual. There is not a problem with graft versus host (GVH) in this procedure.

2. The chemotherapy lowers hematocrit levels, an expected side effect.

3. Low platelets is another expected side effect of chemotherapy. Platelets are the part of our red blood cells that help blood clot.

4. Bone marrow is the spongy tissue found inside your bones. The marrow has a fluid portion where a person's blood cells are developed. This blood cell formation can be examined by use of a bone marrow biopsy and/or by aspiration. Bone marrow aspiration is usually done from the hip bone through a large needle, by which marrow is suctioned out with a syringe. A core biopsy obtains bone marrow with bone fibers. I know Hilary's test required a large needle and syringe, but I don't know if the doctors also obtained bone fibers in the process. After watching the first test in Alaska, I realized this test was surprisingly painful. Hilary was very brave each time I watched the procedure.

5. "Low counts" refers to insufficient quantities of *neutrophils*, the main blood cell that combats infection. Patients with low neutrophil counts do not have a normal immune system to fight even simple infections, so our germ-filled world is too risky for someone with "low counts."

6. Fungi are primitive life forms that we encounter daily. Most are harmless. Candida fungi live in the intestines and mouth, and are kept in check by healthy bacteria living in our bodies. A healthy immune system with healthy bacteria reduces the incidence of harmful fungi. Fungal infections can be difficult to treat, and infected transplant patients have died from them.

7. Platelets are small blood fragments that clot our blood.

8. Receiving a mild case of graft versus host disease (GVHD) allows a graft versus leukemia effect, where lymphocytes will recognize and attack malignant leukemia cells. Unfortunately, too much graft-versus-host will cause the lymphocytes to attack normal tissues, which then causes graft-versus-host disease. This can be deadly.

9. Lynn Eib, *When God and Cancer Meet: True Stories of Hope and Healing* (IL: Tyndale House Publishers, 2002), 175.
10. Annette Mattern, *Outside the Lines* (Texas: Skyward Inc., 2003), ix.
11. J.R.R. Tolkien, *The Lord of the Rings Part One: The Fellowship of the Ring* (New York: Ballantine Publishing Group, 1982), 212.
12. GVHD is caused when the host's (recipient of a donor's stems cells) immune system attack their own tissues. Usually the skin, liver, and gastrointestinal tract are the tissues that GVH injures. The closer a human leukocyte antigen (HLA) matches, the less reaction of GVH.
13. Judith Viorst, *Alexander and the Terrible, Horrible, No Good, Very Bad Day* (New York: Atheneum Books for Young Readers, 1972), 26–27.
14. Mel Gibson, interview by Diane Sawyer, ABC News/Primetime, February 17, 2004, http://abcnews.go.com/Primetime/Oscars2005/story?id=132399&page=1, (accessed January 18, 2010).

ORDER INFORMATION

REDEMPTION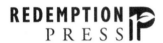
P R E S S

To order additional copies of this book, please visit
www.redemption-press.com.
Also available at Christian bookstores and Barnes and Noble.